POWER FOODS

FOODS

High-Performance Nutrition for High-Performance People

POWER FOODS

High-Performance Nutrition for High-Performance People

by Liz Applegate, Ph.D.

Nutrition Columnist, *RUNNER'S* WORLD Magazine

 RODALE PRESS, EMMAUS, PENNSYLVANIA

Printed in the United States of America on acid-free⊗ paper

Editor: Charles Gerras
Copy Editor: Mary Green   .
Cover and Book Designer: Lisa L. Gatti
Illustrator: Lynn N. Gano
Indexer: Richard Ruane

If you have any questions or comments concerning this book, please write:
      Rodale Press
      Book Reader Service
      33 East Minor Street
      Emmaus, PA 18098

Library of Congress Cataloging-in-Publication Data

Applegate, Elizabeth Ann.
      Power foods : high-performance nutrition for high-performance
people / by Liz Applegate.
            p.   cm.
      Includes index.
      ISBN 0–87857–967–2 hardcover
      1. Nutrition.   I. Title.
RA784.A66   1991
613—dc20   91–16422
                                                         CIP

Distributed in the book trade by St. Martin's Press

   4   6   8   10   9   7   5   hardcover

NOTICE

This book is intended as a reference volume only, not as a medical manual or a guide to self-treatment. If you suspect that you have a medical problem, we urge you to seek competent medical help. Keep in mind that nutritional needs vary from person to person, depending on age, sex, health status, and total diet. The information here is intended to help you make informed decisions about your diet, not to substitute for any treament that may have been prescribed by your doctor.

To Mark, Grant, and Natalie—my loves.

CONTENTS

ACKNOWLEDGMENTS

My deepest thanks to Dr. Paul Kirk, my father, for his editorial and technical guidance and fatherly love. To those seeking to be their best—I thank you for your commitment to excellence. To Kate Delhagen and the gang at *Runner's World,* thanks for your support. Many thanks to Charlie Gerras—a patient and understanding editor; Sarah Enochson for her wonderful typing and organizing; and Russ Suey for his computer wizardry—without him I wouldn't have made it! To my friends—Ann, Cathy, Karen, and Wendy—for their encouragement and warm hearts. To my mother, Marion Kirk, for her loving help, and to my family for their patience. And lastly, to Mark, my husband and friend, for his undying support and love—he made this book possible.

INTRODUCTION

You face challenges daily. Your day is filled with commitments for work, home, and fitness. Instead of your own biorhythms setting the pace, the clock dictates your speed, leaving little time to recover for your next task. Your fast-paced life puts strenuous demands upon your performance and stamina. Ironically, when demands on your performance are the greatest, you literally run out of time to fuel your body properly.

You expect much of your performance, and the stakes are high. But are you performing at your best? Do you have the stamina to keep pace with your expectations? As part of the faster-is-better lifestyle, you must know what, how, and when to fuel your performance and, ultimately, your future. *Power Foods* will show you how to fuel your body for success.

THE POWER FOOD AND PERFORMANCE CONNECTION

Of course, what you eat can profoundly affect the way you feel and look. Athletes and regular exercisers, for instance, have long known the importance of eating a diet high in carbohydrates for better endurance. A low-fat, low-cholesterol diet is standard fare for those fighting off heart disease. But there's more to the power of foods. Did you know that:

- Eating the right foods immediately after a workout or following a hard day at the office will speed your recovery?
- Your eating style may be the cause of your fatigue?
- Certain beverages are better than water in warding off dehydration?
- Properly timed meals may boost your performance at work?

What and how you eat has a powerful influence on your performance. This book will show you how you can optimize body and mind by eating the right foods.

I have counseled many people who want to feel and perform better, just as you do. They talk to me about how drained they feel at the end of the day. The most common requests are, "How can I feel more energetic during a workout?" and "How can I bounce back after a taxing day at work?" I have helped these people—not with elaborate diet plans or special products, but with simple changes in their eating styles and food selections. You'll read about some of these folks and how these changes have helped them. *Power Foods* works for them, now put it to work for you.

In this book, you'll find out about:

□ The ultimate performance 60-15-25 Power Diet and how it can work for your needs.
□ The best beverages for top performance.
□ Your special need for the protein you may not be getting.
□ Which fats *should* be in your diet.
□ The Top Ten Power Foods for super vitamin and mineral nutrition.

There's more of the Power Food/performance connection awaiting you in this book.

THE PLAN

Once you have the facts about Power Foods, it is time for you to personalize a Power-Eating Plan that is specific for your work schedule, exercise habits, and other time constraints. As it is, you have little time left in your day. You certainly don't want to embark on a complicated project. My Power-Eating Plan is designed for you.

I will show you how to meet and conquer daily challenges that would otherwise sap your performance. Find out:

□ How your present eating style rates by taking a simple quiz.
□ What trouble spots you may have in eating style and food selection.
□ Whether you get too few or too many calories.
□ How to lose weight the high-energy way.
□ What to order at restaurants and fast-food outlets for improved stamina.
□ What easy-to-do tactics will help you maintain energy while traveling.
□ How to manage busy home and work schedules in a way that limits fatigue.
□ How to Power Shop at grocery stores.
□ What Power Foods to keep on hand in your kitchen—even if you don't cook.

PART ONE

POWER FOODS: THE FACTS

CHAPTER 1

HIGH-PERFORMANCE DRINKS

Water never ceases to amaze me. It's so simple yet so powerful. As an athlete, you know the revitalizing feeling of drinking cool fluids after a workout. But do you realize how water fuels your everyday work routine? The fatigue, simple headaches, lack of concentration, and dizziness you feel at the end of a workday can result simply from not drinking enough water. What and when you drink affects your stamina and performance.

FLUID NEEDS FOR EVERYDAY PERFORMANCE

Does this scenario sound familiar? It's the end of a long workday and you feel rotten and headachy—your eyes are painfully dry and your whole body has a dull numbness. You blame it on poor sleep over the past few nights and decide to call it a day. Wrong!

Dehydration is most likely your problem. Chances are you drink nothing more than a few cups of coffee in the morning, breathe dry, air-conditioned or heated air at work, and even break into a sweat a few times (that meeting with the boss) during the course of the day—leaving your body parched. As your day goes by, the water lost from your body is not replaced.

Few of my clients think of water as their most important performance ally, when in fact the right amount of water can be the difference between success and failure, on the job as well as during a workout. Understanding water basics—what water does for you and your performance—is necessary so that you can take advantage of this powerful and vital nutrient. Yes, I said "nutrient."

WATER WORKS

You may not think of water as a nutrient, but it is the most critical one in your diet. In fact, you can live only three to four days without water. Virtually every "happening" in your body requires water because it:
☐ Carries the other nutrients throughout the body.
☐ Gives each cell in your body the proper shape and form.
☐ Is essential for maintaining your body temperature.
☐ Lubricates your joints.
☐ Makes food digestion possible.
☐ Rids your body of waste products through the urine.

When your body gets low on fluid, your physical performance and your brain power are impaired. However, when you need to drink some water, your body sends out these early warning signs of dehydration:
☐ Dizziness
☐ Fatigue
☐ Flushed skin
☐ Headache
☐ Impatience
☐ Loss of appetite
☐ Thirst
☐ Weakness

If your body continues to lose water and you fail to take in adequate fluids, matters quickly become more serious. As dehydration progresses, you can expect:
□ Blurred vision
□ Deafness
□ Difficult swallowing
□ Dry, hot, shriveled skin
□ Lack of saliva
□ Rapid pulse
□ Shortness of breath
□ Unsteady gait

Dehydration occurs remarkably often in athletes and hikers not prepared for hot weather. In fact, at one time or another, we all experience mild dehydration, although we may not be aware of it. It taxes our performance and can easily result from skipping a meal, working in dry air, a change in climate, airplane travel, or from *drinking too much coffee or alcohol.*

WATER: WHEREABOUTS AND LOSSES

Somewhere between 50 and 65 percent of your body weight is water—and with all of water's duties, you can see why. For an average-sized man, that's about 96 pints of water, the same volume as 128 cans of soda! However, the more body fat, the less body water you have. The body fat component in women is typically higher than in men, so they tend to have less body water than men (closer to 50 percent of their body weight).

Moreover, not all parts of the body have the same water content, which helps explain why certain body organs suffer more than others when water balance is lost. For example, bone is only about 20 percent water, while blood is virtually all water. Body water depletion quickly manifests itself as reduced blood volume and circulation problems; the bones, however, don't suffer noticeably from dehydration. Since 75 percent of the brain is water, it's no wonder dehydration quickly leads to headaches and dizziness and interferes with its efficiency.

Your body continually loses water as water performs its necessary functions. Every time you exhale, you literally blow off body water—at least two cups per day. Water also evaporates from your skin in order to cool the entire body. Along with

PERCENTAGE OF WATER IN THE HUMAN BODY

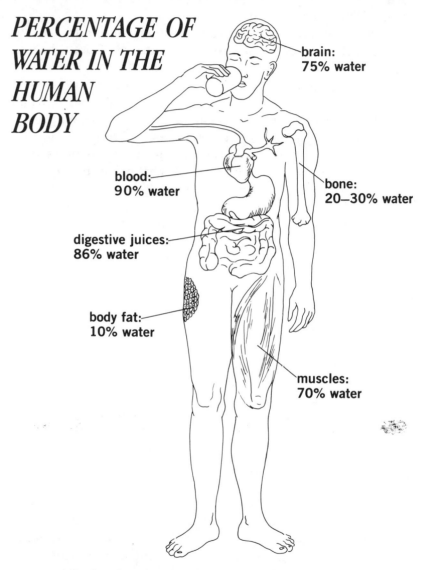

brain:
75% water

blood:
90% water

bone:
20–30% water

digestive juices:
86% water

body fat:
10% water

muscles:
70% water

The average body contains a total of 96 pints of water. Sixty-four pints are found inside the body's cells, with the remainder outside the cells—in the blood, lymph fluid, and digestive juices.

SOURCE: V. Hegarty, *Decisions in Nutrition* (New York: Times Mirror Publishing, 1988).

regular urination and bowel movements, your daily water losses total up to ten cups—not including water lost in sweat, which could double or triple this figure.

Everyday fluid losses go up quickly if you live in a dry climate or at a high altitude, or if you breathe dry air from a heater, dehumidifier, or air conditioner. Plane travel also boosts water loss. Dry air, combined with the rapid circulation of air in a plane, induces even greater loss of water through your skin and from breathing. During a three-hour flight, for example, you could easily lose 1 to 1½ pints of water—the longer the flight, the greater the risk of dehydration. Along with the hectic schedule air travel involves, you may miss a meal or opt for coffee or alcohol, both dehydrating beverages that promote even greater fluid loss, while in flight. How often has flying left you exhausted, irritable, and unable to concentrate? Next time, think about ensuring your water supply in self-defense!

Adding exercise to these water-loss situations dramatically increases body fluid loss. Running, biking, or working out in a gym can easily cost you one to two quarts of fluid per hour. And if you exercise in warm and/or humid weather, water loss jumps up 50 to 100 percent.

Some people perspire more than others when they exercise. Usually, people who are in good shape sweat more, keeping the body cool. Overweight people, however, tend to sweat less, as do children. It's best to get an idea of how much water you lose during a workout by weighing yourself beforehand (without clothes) and again after your workout (dried off and without clothes). Every pound you drop represents a pint of fluid lost. There's more about sweating during exercise and the telltale signs of dehydration later in this chapter.

Beyond exercise and routine daily water losses, other conditions can tax your water balance. Illness, for instance, places a special burden on body water levels. Fever and diarrhea in particular cause large water losses. A simple sunburn also increases water loss, as does weight-loss dieting, because it increases the kidney workload.

There's no way around it—you lose water every minute of every day. The question is, how great are the losses and what's the best way of replacing them? Knowing the precise amount of loss is virtually impossible. You must rely on thirst as your primary guide to fluid intake. When the body loses water, the percentage of water in your blood decreases, making the blood saltier. This draws water out of the mouth and induces thirst.

If you lose water slowly, perhaps during the course of the day in dry air at the office, thirst is a good indicator of your need for fluid replacement, although it is not foolproof. When you lose fluids more quickly, however, such as during exercise, at high altitude, or in situations where several factors affect water loss, thirst is not a reliable indicator of fluid needs. Too often, your sense of thirst is blunted after exercise; some people, such as the elderly, actually have a *decreased* sensation of thirst.

Keep in mind that just being aware of thirst does not remedy dehydration—you have to respond to the signal. Think about the many times you put off getting a drink of water because you were too busy or became distracted. You must make a conscious effort to notice thirst and respond to it ASAP. If you stay attuned to your fluid needs, you will perform better and have more stamina.

Drink beyond your feeling of thirst—one or two additional glasses of fluid—depending upon how rapidly fluid loss occurs. Your body can handle any extra fluid you might consume. Also, basic fluid needs vary, depending upon the situations you face on a particular day. And while you will frequently hear that six to eight glasses of water per day will keep you hydrated, this figure most certainly doesn't hold for those who have heavy sweat losses. Also, it may be excessive for smaller individuals who have modest water losses.

The best guide to your water needs is to observe your urine color and notice how many full bladders of urine you have per day. Your kidneys produce urine to rid the body of unwanted waste from tissues and blood. When urine is a dark yellow color, it means the kidneys were forced to concentrate the waste in a smaller volume of urine. Pale color indicates good hydration status. You should expect a darker shade first thing in the morning, since you haven't been drinking all night. Barring any kidney disease, which can affect urine color and production, you should have at least four full bladders of urine, pale in color, each day. Whether this requires 4 or 12 glasses of water, in addition to

water you consume in the foods you eat, makes no difference—
as long as you drink the water.

FLUID REPLACEMENT HOW-TO

Whether you're struggling with work at your desk or pushing
through a workout at the gym, lost body water means sagging
performance. Yet you constantly face situations that both deplete
your precious body water and interfere with your replenishing
lost fluid. Hectic schedules, skipped meals, exercise, traveling,
weather changes, and long workdays are just a few of the water-
depleting factors you face routinely.

You needn't suffer performance lapses from something as
simple and preventable as dehydration. I'll give you two fluid
replacement guides—one for when you're at work (for routine
water balance control) and one for keeping up with any type of
physical activity. My guides give you simple directions for what,
when, and how much to drink, along with tips you can use to
minimize water loss and optimize filling up.

AT WORK

Even though you're facing work deadlines, changing your daily
routine, breathing in dry, treated air, and drinking dehydrating
beverages, you ask your body to perform at peak levels throughout the day. But your performance is limited by what you drink.
While many causes of fluid loss are out of your control, you are
in control of replacing them. Use these guidelines to do the job.

Start your day with 8 to 16 ounces of water. When you
open your eyes in the morning, your body is already facing a
water deficit (try weighing yourself at night before bedtime and
again in the morning, after voiding, to see how much weight you
lose—water weight, that is). Instead of starting your day off with
a dehydrating cup of coffee or tea, drink a good cup or two of
water, plus a glass of water along with breakfast. Also, keep a
drinking cup in the bathroom so you can sip water while you
ready yourself for the day.

Take water breaks routinely. Whether you are at home, at
work, or out and about, take time for a quick drink of water at

least every 30 to 45 minutes. This will help control any mild dehydration you might suffer due to forgetting to replace your body's fluids for extended periods of time. Drink even more frequently if the air is noticeably dry or hot. The exact amount you should drink depends upon your body size and condition, but ½ cup every hour is a starting point.

Respond to subtle signs of dehydration. Think about drinking fluids as soon as you notice dryness of the eyes, nose, or mouth. Your body is trying to tell you something. These symptoms commonly occur when you breathe dry air, travel, or have a change in climate. Don't put up with even mild discomfort; drink some water right away for consistent performance.

Don't skip meals. When you miss out on breakfast or lunch, you not only cheat yourself on performance nutrients, you also rob your body of water. Much of your daily fluid intake comes during meals—food as well as beverages supply water. Even if you only catch a quick snack, drink fluid along with it.

Avoid dehydrating food and drink. Salty foods temporarily increase your need for water. Your body works to maintain a constant salt concentration in your blood and tissues. Extra salt needs to be diluted with additional water, which eventually will be excreted as urine by the kidneys, whose job is to regulate sodium levels in the body.

Caffeine-containing beverages, like coffee, tea, and some sodas, and alcoholic beverages also change fluid needs. Water losses increase with caffeine, which acts as a diuretic, increasing urine production. (Some people are more affected by caffeine's diuretic action than others.) Drink water along with your morning cup of coffee or tea, or switch to the decaf version. If you drink alcoholic beverages, follow up with a glass or two of water to help replenish lost fluids.

Hydrate well before, during, and after air travel. Thirty to 60 minutes before your flight, drink 8 to 20 ounces of water. This hyperhydration (similar to an athlete's preparation for a workout) helps minimize the dehydrating effects of airplane travel. While aloft, stick with caffeine-free beverages and avoid alcohol, since both may aggravate fluid imbalance. Hold on to your beverage cup on longer flights and ask for refills, or bring a water bottle in your carry-on bag.

Keep fluids readily accessible. You're more apt to keep up with water needs if you keep water and other beverages close at hand. Put a filled water bottle in the glove compartment for your morning commute. Keep a glass of water at your desk and refill it frequently. At home, keep a filled water pitcher in the fridge. Keep a water glass out on the counter as a reminder that you need water.

Recover from schedule changes with proper hydration. When your routine changes—longer work hours, vacation, unscheduled travel—the additional stress may cause you to neglect the signs of dehydration. Use some of the same techniques described above to keep up with fluid losses. Keep in mind that some changes in your daily routine can accelerate fluid losses and that you will need more water than usual to keep performance levels high.

Be aware of weather changes. A rising thermometer means your body has to deal with these warmer temperatures by sweating, to cool off your skin. Feelings of thirst can be delayed when fluid loss is rapid. Make an effort to drink more in warm weather, during travel, and at higher altitudes at any time. The water content of air (humidity) at high altitude is about one-quarter to one-third that of air at sea level, and this causes greater water losses through breathing.

Monitor your sweat losses. You can easily lose large amounts of fluids through sweat during the day, even without exercise. Sudden bursts of effort, like a climb up the stairs or a flurry of activity at work, along with perspiration loss caused by stress or nervousness, can unexpectedly boost water losses. Pay attention to fluid intake on the days you perspire more than usual—your performance can't afford the consequences of dehydration, particularly on these days.

FOR EXERCISE

During exercise—whatever the type—your body generates heat. Dissipating this heat requires fluid evaporation from your skin (sweating), which cools the body. But in an effort to stay cool, your body loses valuable water—anywhere from a few cups with light exercise to one or two quarts an hour during heavy exercise in the heat. As a result, your blood thickens, heart rate goes up, and body temperature starts to climb. Feelings of nausea, headache, chills, and fatigue overtake you, and your performance noticeably deteriorates. In fact, just a 3 percent loss in body weight (4½ pints of sweat during a 90-minute workout) causes a 5 to 10 percent drop in performance.

If water loss continues, symptoms progress to hot, dry skin, disorientation, hallucination, and aggression. You can collapse and even die at this point if water isn't quickly consumed. Working out in hot or humid weather accelerates this process, particularly if you are not acclimated to the weather.

Since dehydration can threaten not only your performance but your life, you need to take action before and during exercise with my simple fluid replacement strategies. During longer workouts, when carbohydrate energy is crucial to your performance, follow the instructions in "Fueling Up after Working Out" on page 20 to optimize fluid and energy replacement.

The following ten steps will keep you going when the heat is on and help you recover quickly to feel great for the rest of the day and through your next workout.

1. Drink up before you exercise. Prepare for upcoming sweat loss by drinking 8 to 20 ounces of water about 15 minutes before working out. For longer exercise sessions, drink more. Avoid starting a workout thirsty. You're destined for substandard performance if you are low on water before you even begin to exercise. Before a competition, make sure you are well hydrated by drinking large amounts of water 24 to 36 hours prior to racing. Look for a pale urine color as a good sign of adequate hydration.

2. During exercise drink frequently. Whether you're training or racing, drink approximately ½ to ¾ cup of water every 10 to 20 minutes. This may seem like a lot, but even this doesn't keep up with typical sweat losses. Experiment with even larger volumes in training, but keep in mind that drinking anything beyond 2 to 2½ quarts in one hour can't be well tolerated. There's a risk of vomiting. Start drinking fluids soon after you've begun the exercise. Waiting until you feel thirsty is too late; chances are you've already lost a fair amount of water.

3. Drink cool fluids. When possible, replenish sweat losses with cool fluids. This helps a bit in cooling your body, and cool fluids also empty out of the stomach faster than warmer beverages, allowing for more rapid fluid absorption. Despite the myths, cold fluids don't cause cramping. Getting cool fluids while you're exercising may be tricky. Keep filled bike bottles in the freezer and take one along for a bike ride, run, or long walk, drinking as it thaws.

4. Stick to water for exercise sessions lasting 60 to 90 minutes, but go for a sport drink for anything longer. You need only water for body cooling and for replenishing losses during shorter exercise. Even though your glycogen (the body's store of carbohydrate) is being used for energy, you have enough to last a good 60 to 90 minutes. Exercise longer than this and you need to take a source of carbohydrate to fuel working muscles and to keep your brain tuned in. (See "Sport Drink Primer" on page 13 and "Fueling Up after Working Out" on page 20 for more specifics on how to use sport drinks.)

5. Drink or eat something with salt during exercise sessions lasting longer than six hours. A pint of sweat contains anywhere from 400 to 2,000 milligrams of sodium (there are 2,000 milligrams of sodium to a teaspoon of salt). If you exercise in hot weather for long periods of time, blood levels of sodium can get dangerously low if you are replenishing only water. Most sport drinks contain ample amounts of sodium for long exercise sessions. Some individuals are at greater risk of suffering from hyponatremia (low blood sodium) during exercise. Eating saltines or pretzels or drinking a soup broth can add needed salt during a lengthy triathlon or run.

If you sweat "gallons," don't be afraid to follow cravings for salt—large amounts lost in sweat need to be replaced. Salt your food moderately during hot-weather training season, but don't overdo, because excessive amounts can pose health risks. And as your body adapts to hot weather, you'll retain more fluid and sodium, which allows you to cool off effectively during exercise.

6. After exercise, quench more than your thirst. Following a workout, your sensation of thirst is not an adequate indicator of how much water you need to balance out losses. Start drinking soon after you finish exercising and plan on drinking at least two to three cups (1 to 1½ pints) beyond quenching your thirst. You should stick to water at first, but sport drinks or carbohydrate-loading beverages can be used to replenish spent carbohydrate as well as lost fluids. Remember to weigh yourself before and after a workout to see how much water you lose during a typical training session.

7. Train yourself to drink wisely and for maximum effect while exercising. During your training sessions, experiment with drinking at regular intervals, try different sport drinks for longer workouts, and play around with different volumes of fluid to see what works best for you. Developing the best fluid replacement strategies during training can improve performance and give you the edge you need in competition.

8. Plan to drink more if you travel to a race. Whether you go by plane, train, or car, traveling dehydrates. Your schedule changes and you may be skipping meals, or at least eating at different times. All of this cheats you of fluids when you can least afford it. Plan on taking a bike bottle filled with water when traveling. Sip from it while you stand in line, wait for a connecting flight, or sit in the car. You'll need extra water if you travel at higher altitudes.

9. Arrive early if you travel to a hot climate. Give yourself about five days to adjust to the high temperatures. Your body will need more water during this time as it adapts by increasing its ability to sweat during exercise. This adaptation allows you to cool off while the heat is on. If you sweat heavily, you may need a little extra salt in your diet to make up for initial losses during adaptation.

10. Avoid drinking concentrated beverages during exercise. You run the risk of further dehydration and stomach upset if you take in beverages like sodas or fruit juices that are more than 10 percent carbohydrate. Above this concentration, water absorption is delayed and body temperature control is impaired. Also, beverages high in fructose (the sugar in fruit juice and some sodas) may cause stomach cramping, bloating, and, potentially, diarrhea.

SPORT DRINK PRIMER

Drinking plain water replaces the volume of lost fluids, but it doesn't replace the energy or electrolytes you need for the long haul. In fact, choosing a sport drink over plain water in some situations can mean success. A good example of this is the performance boost a client of mine had after switching over to an energy replacement drink during his workouts.

Vince, an instructor at a junior college, could fit in two hours of exercise daily after he finished teaching, which was a good four hours after lunch, his last meal. He found himself dragging through his routine on the exercise bike and weights, and many times he simply quit. He took water breaks frequently, so dehydration wasn't his trouble. But when he followed my suggestion to drink about eight ounces of sport drink every 20 to 30 minutes during his workout, Vince couldn't believe the difference in his energy level.

Today's new sport drinks—an array of beverages formulated to replenish fluid and energy spent during exercise—can make a real difference in your workout. In chapter 2, you'll learn that glycogen stores last only so long during exercise—about two hours—before you have to slow down or stop altogether. An incoming supply of carbohydrates is crucial to keep you going, and as pointed out earlier in "Fluid Replacement How-To," salt losses can add up during very long exercise, with serious consequences.

The blend of water, carbohydrate, and electrolytes found in today's sport drinks can replace what exercise drains from you—fluid, fuel, and salt. Recent research shows that, if timed correctly, sport drinks can truly boost your performance. Knowing when to use and how to choose a sport drink will keep you on the winning edge.

Many replacement beverages are on the market today, differing in flavor, carbohydrate type, and concentration. Some contain electrolytes and some even have a dash of added vitamins. The trick is to choose a drink that works for you—tastes good during exercise, doesn't cause intestinal disturbance, and above all, doesn't slow down fluid replacement while supplying carbohydrate energy.

Until a few years ago, available research suggested that sport drinks slowed water's passage into the body, hinting a threat to performance. Sugar concentrations of more than about 3 percent were thought to slow down water absorption and even worsen dehydration. Athletes were frequently advised to water down sport drinks, which are typically 5 to 10 percent carbohydrate, to avoid a performance mishap.

But more recent research shows that it's this theory that should be watered down! Sugar—and the small amount of salt found in today's sport drinks—doesn't slow down water's entry into the bloodstream and may even speed up the process of rehydration. Additionally, weak solutions of carbohydrate, made from watering down a sport drink, provide very little energy for carbohydrate-thirsty muscles.

Experiments with runners, cyclists, and triathletes clearly suggest that carbohydrate solutions ranging from 5 to 10 percent allow for both replenishment of lost water and ample amounts of the carbohydrate energy needed to sustain a long workout or race. In fact, in one such study, cyclists who drank a 6 percent carb solution were able to ride faster after a few hours of pedaling than a group of riders who drank plain water. The sport drink gave these cyclists needed carbohydrate energy to power them in a sprint.

Current research suggests that the ideal carbohydrate concentration should be between 5 and 10 percent. Drinking a beverage above 10 percent, like soda or fruit juice, will slow down water absorption. It also may make you feel nauseated or produce stomach cramps.

CHOOSING A WINNING DRINK

How do you go about choosing the "right" sport drink? Or is there a right drink? Many factors must be considered when choosing a replacement drink, but it's most important that you train with the product and know how to use it. The drinks differ from each other in a number of ways that you should consider when you choose your drink.

Carbohydrate type. There are two categories of carbohydrate: simple sugars, which include glucose, dextrose, fructose, and sucrose (a "double-sugar" of glucose and fructose); and glucose polymers, which are strands of glucose linked together called maltodextrin (often sold under trade names such as Polycose). Your body can use only glucose for its energy needs, but many other carbohydrates are rapidly converted to glucose.

Until recently, researchers recommended glucose-polymer-

POWER FOODS: THE FACTS

Table 1-1 *SPORT DRINK LINEUP*

Product	Calories	Carbohydrate Grams	Carbohydrate Concentration (%)	Electrolytes (mg.) Sodium	Potassium	Calcium	Magnesium
Body Cooler	50	13	6	0	82	75	15
Body Fuel 750	70	17	7	70	20	—	—
Carboplex II	90	22	9	5	—	10	6
Exceed	70	17	7	50	45	—	—
Gatorade	50	14	6	110	25	—	—
Gookinaid E.R.G.	45	12	5	70	100	—	—
Hydra Fuel	66	17	7	25	50	—	—
Paragon High-Performance	50	13	6	55	30	15	6
Performance	100	25	10.5	115	50	40	5
Power Burst	50	13	6	25	50	—	—
Recharge	50	13	6	35	85	—	—
Rehydrate	40	11	4	100	70	—	—
Sudden Impact	70	16	7	94	71	23	—
10-K	56	14	6	54	29	—	—
Workout	80	20	8	30	5	—	—

NOTES: Serving size is 8 ounces.
Data derived from product labels.

containing drinks over simple-sugar sport drinks, since they pass through the stomach more rapidly, potentially allowing for more rapid water absorption. Now it seems that glucose polymers and simple-sugar drinks—in the range of 5 to 10 percent carbohydrate concentration—do equally well at supplying carbohydrate energy while maintaining fluid balance. However, glucose-polymer drinks don't taste as sweet as sugared beverages. This means you can drink more carbohydrate in the form of glucose polymer without that sticky-sweet aftertaste.

You should avoid drinks high in fructose. This simple sugar, found in sodas and fruit juices, can bring on nausea and diarrhea at a concentration of 10 percent or more. Most other simple-sugar beverages are tolerated well at 10 percent concentration and even a little beyond, while glucose-polymer drinks sit well in some athletes up to about 15 percent carbohydrate concentration.

Electrolyte addition. Replacement beverages may also have added electrolytes—sodium, potassium, magnesium, and calcium—which may improve the taste and lead to increased fluid consumption. But there is an added advantage of electrolyte addition to sport drinks. Small amounts of sodium improve water and glucose absorption into the body. In fact, glucose/electrolyte drinks have been shown to maintain body-fluid balance better than glucose drinks alone.

For the most part, electrolytes don't need to be replaced during exercise, since salt losses are replenished quite adequately in the diet. However, in extreme situations, electrolyte depletion does occur during long sessions of exercise. This problem of salt depletion, or hyponatremia, is not a common one, but a number of ultra-endurance athletes have experienced this condition during the Ironman Triathlon in Hawaii and other endurance events.

Sport drinks that contain sodium range from 50 to just over 100 milligrams of sodium per cup (about the amount in half a bagel). Sweat contains from 400 to 2,000 milligrams of sodium per pint. Sodium content in sweat depends upon many factors, but as you become more fit and sweat even more, the concentration of sodium drops.

Flavor. Yes, the flavor can affect your performance—indirectly that is. Whether the drink is orange, mixed citrus, or fruit-punch flavor can influence how much of it you are willing to drink. Carbohydrate-sweetened drinks lead to greater fluid consumption than plain water. If the taste makes you drink more, you stay better hydrated. When it comes to fruit punch over lemon-lime, or vice versa, that's up to you. Some people like a change in flavor from time to time, and this may help your "compliance."

The point is, don't use a sport drink that doesn't taste good to you. Since our tastes differ, try a number of products to get a sampling of what they are like. If you plan to use a sport drink in competition, try it out in training so you don't get any surprises come race day.

WATER PRIMER

If you're like a growing number of health-seeking Americans, you are turning off tap water and downing bottled water in the hope of getting a more healthful and better-tasting drink. In 1990 alone, Americans quenched their thirst with more than $2 billion worth of bottled water. But are they getting what they are paying for? Sometimes ... that is, sometimes bottled waters are more healthful than tap water, but don't count on it. Understanding tap water safety regulations, and learning to decipher bottled water lingo, will help you choose the best water to quench your thirst.

TAP WATER SAFETY

The list of possible contaminants in drinking water from the tap reads like a roll call for a hazardous waste dump. How safe your tap water is depends upon where you live, but statistics from the Environmental Protection Agency (EPA), the government agency charged with ensuring safe drinking water, suggest that about one-fifth of the nation's community water supply does not meet safety standards. Tap water can be contaminated with bacteria, cancer-causing chemicals like trihalomethanes (coming from chlorine used in treating water), radioactive radon, and a host of other pollutants.

The EPA requires that your water provider test regularly for contaminants—about 80 of them. You can get the results of this water testing simply by calling your community water works. Once you find out how much of what contaminant is in your water, you can then call the EPA Safe Drinking Water Hotline (1-800-426-4791) to learn if these levels are too high and what guidelines there may be for contaminants that have no official standards.

If your water supply comes from a private well, you should consider testing your tap water if you notice a change in odor, color, or taste; if you live near underground gasoline tanks or a hazardous waste dump; or if you suspect the presence of lead from water pipes. Do-it-yourself water testing kits are available at some supermarkets and hardware stores for about $10 to $15; if you prefer to have a professional evaluation, call the EPA hotline for the name of a registered laboratory in your state.

All this contamination talk probably has put tap water on your list of no-no's. But there are some elements in tap water that are actually quite healthful. Minerals, which give water its taste (good or bad), are found in fairly high levels in some water supplies. Hard water contains relatively high concentrations of minerals like calcium and magnesium. Soft water has very little of these minerals, but instead has higher levels of sodium.

In areas with naturally hard water, many households opt to soften the water by removing the calcium and magnesium. This reduces the buildup of deposits on faucets and allows soaps and shampoos to do their thing. However, sodium replaces calcium and magnesium during the softening process, which can boost sodium intake beyond desirable levels for those people with high blood pressure. On the average, drinking water supplies 10 percent of your total sodium intake. But for people on restricted sodium diets, drinking water may account for 64 percent of total sodium intake.

You can relieve some of your concern about tap water safety with the installation of a filtering device on your faucet. These filtering systems, designed to remove major contaminants such as trichloromethanes, run from $30 to over $500. Their performance can vary just as much as their price, but price is not a sure indicator of quality. Before you buy, check with the manufacturer to see if the product has been EPA-tested, and ask how well the major pollutants are removed.

FUELING UP AFTER WORKING OUT

Whether you're doing your regular workout or setting your eyes on competition, how you refuel can mean success or failure. I've put it all together in the refueling plan below, which outlines how much water, sport drink, or solid food to eat depending upon the length of your workout or competition.

Use this guide to get you started on successful refueling. You're the best judge of how much water and energy replacement you need for different workouts. Keep track of how you feel with different refueling techniques: how much, what, and how often you drink, and what you eat. You may find, early into your exercise program, that you can eat or drink more without discomfort, or you may notice that you can eat only solid foods during cycling but not during running. As you gain experience with refueling, you will find greater success in your workouts and competition.

Table 1-2 *REFUELING GUIDE*

Duration of Exercise	Water	Sport Drink	Solid Food
Less than 1 hour	½ cup at 30 min.	None required	None required
1–2 hours	½–¾ cup every 10–15 min. plus solid food	Most often not needed, but ½–1 cup total may help some people	None required; or small piece of fruit like orange slice
2–4 hours	Same as 1–2 hours if only solid foods eaten	¾ cup every 10–20 min.	75–150 calories every 30 min.

(continued)

Table 1-2—*Continued*

Duration of Exercise	Water	Sport Drink	Solid Food
4–6 hours	Same as 1–2 hours if only solid foods eaten	¾ cup every 20 min; use beverage with sodium	75–150 calories every 30 min.; include foods with sodium: breads, crackers, cookies

SOURCE: Adapted in part from W. Mike Sherman and D.R. Lamb, "Nutrition and Prolonged Exercise," *Prolonged Exercise* (Carmel, Ind.: Benchmark Press, 1988), 213–80.

BOTTLED H₂O

About one out of every six households is turning to bottled water as its primary source of drinking water—the number is twice that in California. A major reason cited by most consumers for turning off the tap and opening a bottle is doubt about tap water safety. However, just because water is sold in slick bottles with fancy labels doesn't mean that it is any safer than the water that comes straight out of your faucet. Depending upon the type of bottled water, fewer safety regulations may apply than for tap water. Equip yourself with a little bottled water savvy before you shop for packaged water.

A quick glance at the beverage aisle in your supermarket will convince you that the world of specialty waters is a confusing one. A few definitions may help you understand exactly what it is you're swallowing.

Still water or drinking water is noncarbonated and typically used as an alternative to tap water. More than 90 percent of bottled water sales are for still water. The source is variable and may well be the municipal water supply, not necessarily a well or spring.

Sparkling water has carbon dioxide introduced to make it bubbly, and *naturally sparkling water* has enough carbon dioxide occurring naturally in the water source to give it fizz.

Distilled water has been vaporized and condensed and therefore contains no minerals. (It may not be free of microorganisms or organics sloughed off from ion-exchange purifiers.)

Spring water flows out of the earth, is bottled near its source, and is not altered by the addition or deletion of minerals or carbonation.

Mineral water contains a variety of minerals, predominantly calcium, magnesium, and sodium, naturally present in the water source. Mineral content varies depending upon the source, but virtually all waters, with the exception of distilled and purified water, contain some minerals. The International Bottled Water Association, however, states that mineral waters must contain not less than 500 parts per million total dissolved solids (minerals and salts). Mineral waters may or may not fizz.

Seltzer is usually plain old tap water with added fizz, but no added minerals. Many seltzers have added sweeteners like corn syrup or sucrose. So unlike other bottled waters, seltzers are not necessarily calorie-free.

Club soda is artificially carbonated tap water with added minerals and salts.

Interestingly, bottled water has to meet fewer safety standards for contaminants than tap water. Also, mineral waters, seltzers, club soda, and naturally sparkling waters are considered under the same safety testing category as soft drinks. This means they are tested for even fewer potential contaminants and are allowed to have additives such as caffeine and alcohol. However, bottlers routinely check for contaminants, and you can request the most recent results to check for safety.

Mineral waters, depending upon the brand, may contain a reasonable amount of minerals such as magnesium and calcium. While your diet supplies a majority of these nutrients from foods like green leafy vegetables and dairy products, you may not be getting enough. Magnesium, for instance, is a very important mineral for everyday performance and exercise (see chapter 5), but some 40 percent of all Americans get insufficient amounts from their diet. Vittel mineral water supplies 100 percent of the

U.S. Recommended Daily Allowance (USRDA) for this mineral in one liter.

Check Table 1-3 for mineral water profiles. Remember, however, that virtually all water contains some minerals. Ask your local water company for an index of water hardness (an indication of mineral content). Some local water supplies have calcium and magnesium levels higher than those in some bottled mineral waters. You can expect to pick up something in the way of minerals by drinking any type of water—bottled or tap—except for "distilled" or "purified" water.

So is bottled better? Some bottled waters are definitely better than the tap option; others are not. The best way for you to settle this water source dilemma in your own mind is to check out the purity of the product your faucet supplies. If you can tolerate the taste of your tap water and it's "clean" of contaminants, then drink up . . . it's free.

MORE DRINK OPTIONS

You probably have a good idea by now that your body needs quality fluid replacement. But that's not what it usually gets. Consumption of plain water has gone down over the past 20 years, and use of water alternatives, like soft drinks, is going up rapidly. While sodas, coffee, beer, fruit drinks, and other fluid concoctions are mostly water, they present your body with some not-so-healthy extras like acids, caffeine, and alcohol. These water alternatives also detract from your nutrient intake by substituting for more nutritious fluids like fruit or vegetable juices.

Below I outline some facts you should know about the two most commonly used water alternatives: soft drinks and coffee. This information, along with bottled water basics, will help you choose the right thirst quencher and fluid replacement for everyday performance.

HARD FACTS ON SOFT DRINKS

Believe it or not, we drink more soda than tap water. Back in 1964, every American averaged over 72 gallons a year from the tap and 17 gallons a year of soda. But now, each of us gulps down over 42 gallons of fizzy fluid (diet and regular) annually, and only 41 gallons of tap water. And it looks as though we will keep

Table 1-3 *WHAT'S IN THE BOTTLE?*

Product	Mineral Content (mg/l)		
	Calcium	Magnesium	Sodium
Mineral Waters			
Asante	trace	trace	187
Calistoga	1	1	151
Crystal Geyser	2	1	167
La Croix	27	trace	1
Perrier	128	2	6
Vittel	32	364	9
Seltzers			
Koala	94	55	110
Old San Francisco	36	5	31
Original New York	10	6	11
Sundance	28	48	67
Spring and Sparkling Waters			
Evian	78	24	5
Oasis	51	10	16
Poland	11	1	1

NOTE: Data derived from product labels.

drinking more soda and less water with every passing year—as we have over the last 20 years. However, such a passion for sodas is not without risk.

If you are one of the many who average more than 16 ounces a day of soda, consider the following when you are quenching your thirst with this water alternative.

Sugared sodas are the most popular type. They supply about 160 calories of sugar per 12-ounce can and nothing else in the way of nutrients. Fruit juice has the same amount of sugar from fruit, but it also provides some vitamins and minerals for performance. Not only is a sugared soda missing key nutrients, but the high sugar content promotes tooth decay at any age.

Soda often takes the place of milk at mealtime. This is particularly the case for children and teenagers. This means that much-needed calcium is being preempted and more calcium may even be lost from the body when we drink certain sodas. Typically, dark-colored sodas contain phosphoric acid, which can upset the calcium balance in the body. The phosphorus increases calcium loss in the urine if calcium intake is low.

Soft drink enthusiasts average much less than their requirement of calcium. Also, we don't have a generation of older people yet who have grown up on soft drinks, as today's teenagers have, so we don't know what this habit will do to their bone health in later years. Clearly, the increasing trend of drinking a soda instead of milk for breakfast is not a healthful one.

Many sodas contain caffeine. You certainly don't get this additive from tap water. While the amount of caffeine in one 12-ounce can of soda is about half that of a cup of coffee (see "Caffeine Stats" on page 29), heavy soda drinkers and children may be getting too much. Caffeine is a stimulant that increases feelings of alertness, but it also acts as a diuretic, increasing fluid loss through the urine. Quenching your thirst with a caffeine-type soda doesn't make sense, since it actually increases your fluid needs.

Sugar-free sodas may indeed save you calories. However, these drinks still may contain caffeine and phosphoric acid, so check the label for these ingredients. If you're working on your third or fourth soda of the day, switch over to a caffeine-free variety, and a light-colored one that contains no phosphorus. Better yet, try water with a twist of lime. Also, using sugar-free sodas does not mean you will lose weight. The consumption of artificially sweetened sodas is up dramatically, but Americans are not getting any thinner. (See "Sweetening Artificially" on page 81 for more about these sweeteners.)

"Naturally" sweetened sodas contain refined sugar. Many of these products claim to have no refined sugar or additives, such as caffeine or artificial colors or flavors. Yet, the "natural" sugar from fruit juice is fructose, which is a refined sugar. Fructose can cause elevated blood fat levels in susceptible people.

The natural flavors do not have any nutritional advantage, but they may give the soda a better taste.

COFFEE CONTROVERSY

Do you find yourself sipping your morning coffee with some reservation? Should you join the growing caffeine-free generation to avoid the many suspected health risks? Research over the last ten years has linked coffee or caffeine to cancer, breast disease in women, heart disease, and digestive problems, to name a few. Such news has led to a steady decline in coffee consumption. We now average 1.6 cups of java daily, compared with 3.1 cups in 1962.

However, despite the bad news, some 50 percent of American adults still drink coffee, and an untold percentage gulp down caffeinated sodas, mostly for caffeine's performance-enhancing ability to perk up mood, alertness, and possibly endurance. If you're a coffee or cola lover, don't despair. You can sip with a sigh of relief—new research suggests caffeine may not be all bad.

For instance, there is good news for people trying to control their weight and for those suffering from asthma. Also, recent research sheds some doubt on coffee's link to cancer, heart disease, and other disorders. But there's not-so-good news for coffee-drinking women trying to conceive. To help sort out the hot and cold on coffee and caffeine, consider the following:

Heart disease. Should coffee be added to the list of no-no's for people trying to avoid heart disease and to lower blood cholesterol? The Surgeon General feels that present research is insufficient to make a recommendation to give up coffee drinking. However, a number of studies have demonstrated a link between heavy coffee drinking and a greater incidence of heart disease. For instance, a Johns Hopkins Medical Institution study that followed 1,130 male medical students over a 19- to 35-year period found that those who drank five or more cups per day were over two times more likely than others to develop coronary heart disease.

However, a problem with this study and others is the possible differences in diet and lifestyle between heavy coffee drinkers and those who avoid coffee. While the researchers from Johns

Hopkins did account for smoking and a few other heart-disease-related risk factors, they did not take into account the type of diet each man ate over the years. The heavy coffee drinkers, for example, might have eaten a riskier high-fat diet, explaining their increased likelihood to develop heart disease.

Studies linking caffeine to elevated blood cholesterol levels are also inconsistent. In fact, caffeine may not be responsible for boosting this artery-clogging fat; instead it may be the way coffee is brewed or a substance in coffee other than caffeine. One study involving over 9,000 men and women found high blood cholesterol was linked with coffee consumption but not with total caffeine intake from other sources like tea and cola.

Researchers from Norway have proposed that brewing methods might explain higher blood cholesterol levels. More than 18,000 men and women were interviewed about coffee use, brewing methods, and diet. Cholesterol levels tended to climb with greater coffee use in those individuals who drank boiled coffee, but not in people using such other brewing methods as filtering. The researchers propose that a yet-to-be-identified substance in coffee affects metabolism of cholesterol and that the length of time the coffee grounds are in hot water influences the amount or action of this mystery substance.

Cancer and breast disease. Reports from several years ago put coffee on the ever-growing cancer-causing list. But subsequent reports, even by the same researchers who linked coffee to cancer, refute this connection. Presently there is no strong evidence to link regular coffee drinking with any form of cancer. For instance, a study that attempted to relate coffee and tea drinking in women from 44 countries with the rate of death from breast cancer found no relationship.

However, fibrocystic breast disease in women, a noncancerous and benign disorder, does appear to have a possible link with coffee consumption. While results are somewhat confusing, these breast lumps appear to be more common in women who are heavy coffee drinkers—four- or five-plus cups daily. One study showed a small reduction in lump size when women abstained from caffeine, but it is not clear whether this is of clinical significance, and other studies have not supported these results.

Obesity and weight control. Encouraging research findings suggest the amount of caffeine in one cup of coffee can boost the number of calories you burn while resting (basal metabolic rate). When subjects were given 100 milligrams of caffeine (equivalent to a cup of coffee) every 2 hours for a 12-hour period, resting energy expenditure went up 8 to 11 percent. Also, researchers found that caffeine given to overweight people boosted the amount of energy they burned after eating a meal. Unlike normal-weight individuals, some obese people typically don't increase energy expenditure after a meal. These results show some promise in treating the problem of depressed energy expenditure in obese individuals and, perhaps, in promoting weight loss.

Asthma. Daily coffee consumption may also reduce the risk of developing asthma. A survey of more than 70,000 adults reveals that those individuals drinking up to three cups per day experience 27 fewer cases of bronchial asthma than people who do not drink any coffee. A reduced risk of asthma was also seen in those drinking just one cup per day. While past research shows asthma symptoms decrease with caffeine intake (because it acts much like a commonly used asthma drug), this study suggests a protective effect from coffee.

Fertility and pregnancy. Not all the news brewing with coffee is good. A study involving 104 healthy women attempting to become pregnant suggests coffee might have a negative effect on fertility. The women who drank one cup of coffee per day were half as likely to become pregnant as women who drank less. And the more coffee the women drank, the less likely they were to conceive during the three-month study period. More research is needed to verify these results, but couples interested in having children may want to slow their coffee consumption.

Pregnant women also may want to cut back on caffeine intake. A study with over 3,000 pregnant women found those consuming the amount of caffeine in three cups of coffee had more than 4.5 times the risk of delivering a low-birth-weight infant, which increases the risk for infant mortality. The rate of processing caffeine in a pregnant woman is three times slower than that in a nonpregnant woman.

Additionally, a baby has no ability to metabolize caffeine until several days after birth, which may account for the irregular heartbeat seen in newborns from mothers who took in over 300 milligrams of caffeine just before giving birth. This evidence suggests caffeine may slow the growth of a developing fetus and may have transitory effects on the newborn. Until more research is done, pregnant women should curb caffeine intake from coffee, tea, and sodas. (See "Caffeine Stats" below.)

Performance. It's not hot news that caffeine is a quick pick-me-up any time of day, but can an afternoon cola or cup of brew really improve your physical or mental performance? The amount of caffeine in one to two cups of brewed coffee increases

CAFFEINE STATS

Effects of 200 milligrams of caffeine on the body:
□ Increases alertness and reduces fatigue
□ Increases urine flow
□ Stimulates stomach acid secretion
□ Increases heartbeat and blood pressure temporarily
□ Interferes with sleep

Peak acting time: 30 to 60 minutes after ingestion.

Half-life: Approximately half of a caffeine dose is cleared from the body after 3½ hours, and after 12 hours all of the dose is metabolized. Smokers process caffeine faster, and pregnant women, children, and the elderly clear caffeine more slowly, taking up to 72 hours.

Side effects of intakes over 300 to 1,000 milligrams (depending on the person):
□ Insomnia
□ Shaking and nervousness
□ Irregular heartbeats
□ Increased breathing
□ Enhanced feelings of anxiety

Lethal dose: 10,000 milligrams, the amount in 100 cups of coffee consumed during a 30-minute period.

feelings of alertness and reduces fatigue and drowsiness in most people. Caffeine also speeds up your reaction time, but there is no evidence that caffeine improves your thinking ability beyond keeping you awake.

A dose of caffeine before exercise has been shown to enhance performance for some people, but not everyone. Besides acting as a stimulant, caffeine also hastens muscle contraction. And during endurance exercise it promotes fat use for energy, sparing precious muscle glycogen. Various studies demonstrate that athletes can run or cycle longer following caffeine ingestion equivalent to the amount in three cups of coffee. Yet an equal number of studies show that caffeine has no positive effect on endurance.

Getting a boost out of caffeine appears to depend upon how regularly you consume coffee, tea, or cola. Habitual coffee drinkers develop a tolerance to caffeine. This means the typical side effects, like rapid heart rate, increased urine production, and

CAFFEINE CONTENT OF COMMON PRODUCTS

Brewed coffee, 1 cup: 50–150 milligrams
Instant coffee, 1 cup: 30–120 milligrams
Sweetened coffee mix, General Foods:
    40–80 milligrams
Decaffeinated coffee, 1 cup: 2–8 milligrams
Brewed tea, 1 cup: 20–100 milligrams
Instant tea, 1 cup: 30–70 milligrams
Colas, 12 ounces: 36–46 milligrams
Mountain Dew, 12 ounces: 54 milligrams
Hot cocoa, 1 cup: 4–8 milligrams
Semisweet chocolate, 1 ounce: 14 milligrams
Excedrin, 2 tablets: 130 milligrams
Vivarin, 1 tablet: 200 milligrams
Nō-Dōz, 1 tablet: 100 milligrams

SOURCE: Adapted from J.A.T. Pennington, *Bowes and Church's Food Values of Portions Commonly Used,* 15th ed. (Philadelphia: J. B. Lippincott, 1989).

nervousness, are reduced. Developing a tolerance also appears to desensitize the body to caffeine's positive effects during exercise.

A study examined the effect of caffeine dosing before exercise in coffee-drinking athletes who had abstained from caffeine for four days. The caffeine boosted their blood levels of free fatty acids, which are used for energy during exercise, more following the withdrawal period than when the athletes stuck to their regular caffeine habit. These results suggest that glycogen sparing and enhanced performance from a caffeine dose would be more likely in a "caffeine-free" body. Caffeine may lose its punch as a performance enhancer if it's a staple in your diet.

Last drop. Does all this mean you should give up your daily coffee or cola? Hardly. If you drink moderate amounts of coffee—two cups daily—you benefit safely from caffeine's wake-up appeal. However, if you're plagued with symptoms of "coffee nerves," have problems with irregular heartbeats (which caffeine may aggravate), or find yourself "hydrating" with coffee or caffeinated colas all day long—cut back and see if your symptoms improve.

CHAPTER **2**

CARBOHYDRATE:
the ultimate performance food

Michael glances frantically at the time—it's four o'clock, and with at least three more hours of paperwork to do, the desire for an after-work run is fading. "I just don't have the energy to keep this up," he complains to himself (it's the third night this week Michael has given up his workout because of fatigue). Both the problem and the solution stem from the type and quantity of carbohydrates Michael eats.

Even though Cindy's schedule is packed to the limit—a part-time teaching job plus raising two boys—she is determined to enter her first 10-K run next month. But Cindy is beginning to doubt her ability to make the run. Each time she trains for three consecutive days she feels completely drained, and on the fourth day,

Cindy gives up her training routine until the following week. Her diet history reveals that her evening meals typically consist of cheese and crackers and wine eaten while preparing dinner for her family. Cindy's problem, like Michael's, is a carbohydrate deficit—not enough of the right fuel to get her through a demanding schedule.

THE HIGH-CARBOHYDRATE DIET: PERFORMANCE FUEL

Your performance highs (and lows) center around the superfuel food: carbohydrate—the most important nutrient for achieving peak stamina. Whether you are pushing to finish those last miles of your run or surviving a long day at the office, a diet loaded with carbohydrate foods is a must. I will show you a simple plan for powering your performance with carbohydrate.

First, let's understand why carbohydrate is so vital as the brain fuel you use for thinking power, as well as the muscle fuel you use for physical power. By physical power I mean running a 10-K, running through airports, or having the stamina to give a crisp, dynamic four-hour presentation to your clients. You simply need to know when, how much, and what type of carbohydrates to eat.

FOOD CARBOHYDRATES

Affectionately called "carbs" by athletes, carbohydrates are divided into two categories. The first group consists of simple carbohydrates, made from one or two ring-shaped molecules called sugar units. The second group is complex carbohydrates, a large chain of simple sugar units. Both simple and complex carbohydrates occur in foods such as grains, fruits, and vegetables.

Simple carbs circulate in your blood and are appropriately called blood sugar. Your body's basic sugar unit is called glucose, and while there are other types of sugars (see "Sugars: Types and Sources" on page 34), glucose plays the major role in supplying your mind and body with power. Since your body's metabolic machinery can't make enough glucose, you must get it from the foods you eat. If you're like most of those who seek top performance, you're probably not getting enough of this power nutrient from your diet.

Simple carbohydrates are the hallmark of the American diet and are found in many of the foods we eat—processed and natural. Chemically speaking, the simple carbohydrates are called monosaccharides (a single sugar unit) and disaccharides (two sugar units linked together). Simple carbohydrates abound in foods like table sugar and honey (which are virtually pure simple sugar) and in foods that have added sugar, like cookies, candy, and other sweet-tasting goodies. Fruit is also loaded with simple sugars, primarily a monosaccharide called fructose. Simple carbohydrates also pop up in places you might not expect, like milk (which contains lactose, a disaccharide), and beer (which contains maltose, another disaccharide).

Sugars, by virtue of their chemical structure, taste . . . well, great. I mean sweet. And that's just it! Sugars taste too good to most of us, and consequently we gobble down sugary foods at too high a rate (125 pounds of sugar per person per year, the amount in over 10,000 cookies!). The primary health concern with this high sugar consumption is malnutrition. Most high-

SUGARS: TYPES AND SOURCES

Fructose: Found in fruits and honey, fructose is added to foods, particularly sodas, as a sweetener.

Galactose: This is found in milk as part of lactose.

Glucose: Found in fruits, glucose is added to foods as a sweetener. In the body, it is called blood sugar.

Lactose: Found in milk, lactose is a sugar made of glucose and galactose.

Maltose: Found in sprouted seeds and beer, maltose is the result of starch breakdown. It is often added to processed foods.

Sucrose: This is common table sugar, added as a sweetener, and is made up of glucose and fructose.

sugar food (with the exception of milk and sprouted seeds) is a nutritional void, providing little in the way of needed nutrients for optimal health. But you can and should satisfy your natural desire for sweet-tasting foods. (See "Eat Sweets the Right Way" later in this chapter for more on eating sweets without worrying about nutritional mishaps.)

Complex carbohydrates, on the other hand, don't have the sweet reputation of simple carbohydrates, even though they are nothing more than a chain of simple sugar units of glucose. The most common complex carbohydrate is called starch, a molecule that is made up of many (hundreds) of glucose units linked together. It looks like a string of Christmas lights when seen through a powerful microscope. This string of glucose units represents a major source of food energy for most of us. Starch, found in dried beans, vegetables, fruit, and grains like wheat and rice, is easily broken down in your digestive tract into glucose. Your body then moves the glucose units to wherever they are needed—muscles, brain, liver—where glucose can be used for energy or stored for later use.

Another benefit of eating complex carbohydrates is that you get a good amount of fiber. One type of fiber, cellulose, simply passes through the digestive tract. Even though it is resistant to digestion, it plays a vital role in keeping your digestive tract healthy by "toning" the intestines and preventing constipation. Also, fiber may help in preventing certain types of intestinal cancer and, in certain situations, may aid in weight loss. For a carbohydrate that doesn't get inside the body's metabolism, fiber certainly is vital for our health and performance.

BODY CARBOHYDRATES

Another complex carbohydrate, glycogen, occurs exclusively in the body, never in food. Glycogen serves as a reservoir of carbohydrate that your body can use for energy. Microscopically similar to the starch molecule in a slice of bread, the glycogen molecule is packed away in the muscles and liver for those times when you need energy. Glycogen in the muscles is broken down to glucose units and supplies energy during exercise and quick bursts of muscle activity, like sprinting to catch the bus. Glycogen in the liver offers glucose on demand, via the bloodstream, to all organs and tissues—most important, to the brain, keeping it alert and functioning smoothly.

Whether you eat a sugary candy bar which is mostly simple carbohydrates or a baked potato loaded with complex carbohydrates, the end-product carbohydrate flowing through your body and stored in your muscle is the simple sugar, glucose—the basic energy currency in the body.

The job of breaking down complex carbohydrates in food is handled by your intestines. This digestive process happens almost instantaneously for simple sugars because, in effect, they are so refined they are already "digested." For that reason, simple carbohydrates pass into your bloodstream more rapidly than complex carbohydrates. In other words, the carbohydrate in the fruit or candy bar you eat moves into your system faster than the same amount of carbohydrate you get from a baked potato. But once inside the body, glucose fuels your performance throughout the day, regardless of the speed with which it enters the body from your food.

The choice you make between simple and complex carbohydrate foods has a profound impact on your health and performance. Even though they both provide needed glucose, complex carbohydrates provide several nutritional advantages, such as additional vitamins, minerals, and fiber needed for good health and performance. (For more on sugars and your health, see "Sweetness: Real, Artificial, or None at All?" on page 74.)

WHY CARBOHYDRATES FOR PERFORMANCE?

There is a simple way to address that question by reflecting on your own experience. Have you ever:

☐ Felt tired, listless, unable to concentrate midmorning or late afternoon?

☐ Started a workout but quit partway through because you were too tired and weak to finish?

☐ Found yourself in the middle of a long training run or race and you simply couldn't keep up the pace the way you could at other times?

◻ Entertained the thought of giving up your exercise routine altogether in the hope that you would have more energy to use at work and home?

Yes, yes, yes, and yes. Who hasn't felt tired at some time or another? But for many of us, inadequate dietary carbohydrate is the culprit, and for good reason. The amount and kind of carbohydrates you eat directly influence how much glucose (carbohydrate) you have in your blood and how much is stored as glycogen in your muscles and liver. This is what I call "body carbohydrate," and it affects your well-being and performance most profoundly.

A certain amount of glucose must be maintained in the blood to keep you feeling alert and healthy. If your blood glucose falls below normal, you become shaky, tired, and hungry; if the blood glucose level goes too high, you can become sleepy and even run the risk of a coma. Luckily, a very elegant system of hormone balancing usually acts to control your blood glucose level. Optimal blood glucose level is most important for clear, smooth brain function and is therefore critical to sharp, high-speed mental performance. Your eating habits can undermine or enhance how well your blood sugar level is controlled and, hence, how you feel and perform.

CARBS FOR BRAIN POWER

For the most part, your body keeps blood sugar levels normal throughout the day and night, but sporadic eating patterns can hinder your body's best efforts. If you skip a meal, breakfast for instance, your body has to draw on the liver's supply of glycogen for energy. This supply eventually runs low, and your blood sugar level begins to drop, giving you a hungry, tired feeling. This lowering of fuel supply to the brain can have a negative effect on your mental power.

Studies show that memory, reaction time, and performance on proficiency tests are diminished in people who skip their morning meal. It probably doesn't surprise you, then, that on those days you rush out without eating in the morning, your day at the office is less productive. Regular breakfast skippers are convinced this style of eating is best for them. Yet they always find their alertness and productivity improve when they try a light morning meal of cereal and milk or fruit and toast.

Skipping your midday meal can also affect your mental performance, particularly when you have missed breakfast. Your brain is unable to store the energy it needs to keep functioning, so it is essential that you eat with some regularity. Hit-or-miss eating patterns—skipping breakfast one day, missing out on lunch the next, or missing both breakfast and lunch—can pull your gray matter into a temporary state of slow motion.

TOP COMPLEX-
CARBOHYDRATE FOODS

Breads and Crackers
- Bagels (all types)
- Crackers (soda, RyKrisp, Ak-Mak)
- Multigrain breads, sprouted-grain breads
- Pita bread
- Pretzels
- Rolls (dinner type, hamburger, etc.)
- Rye, pumpernickel bread
- Tortilla (corn, flour)
- Whole-wheat and white bread

Cereals
- Grits (cooked, plain)
- Oatmeal, oat bran cereal
- Puffed cereal (rice, corn, or multigrain)
- Ready-to-eat, low-sugar types (e.g., bran flakes, shredded wheat)
- Wheat germ
- Whole-grain cooked cereal

Dried Beans
- Baked beans (no added meat)
- Black-eyed peas
- Kidney, pinto, navy beans
- Lentils
- Split peas

(continued)

Top Foods—*Continued*

Fruits (also contain simple sugars)

- Apples
- Apricots
- Bananas
- Berries
- Cantaloupe
- Cherries
- Dried fruit
- Figs
- Grapefruit
- Grapes
- Kiwis
- Nectarines
- Oranges
- Papayas
- Peaches
- Pears
- Pineapple
- Plums
- Strawberries
- Watermelon

Grains

- Barley
- Rice, brown and white
- Wheat bulgur
- Other cooked grains: quinoa, amaranth, millet

Pasta

- All types (cooked, plain)

Starchy Vegetables

- Corn
- Lima beans
- Peas
- Potatoes (white and red)
- Sweet potatoes and yams
- Winter squash (acorn, butternut, spaghetti)

Vegetables

- Artichokes
- Asparagus
- Beans (green)
- Beets
- Broccoli
- Cabbage
- Carrots
- Chard
- Kale
- Leeks
- Lettuce (all types)
- Mushrooms
- Onions
- Peppers (red, green)
- Rutabaga
- Spinach
- Squash
- Tomatoes
- Turnip greens
- Vegetable juice

FEED YOUR MUSCLES

Besides your brain's needing carbohydrates for mental energy, the rest of your body also relies heavily on glucose for power. Your muscles are the major consumers of carbohydrate energy. When you are inactive—sitting, lying down, or sleeping—only small amounts of carbohydrates are used for energy (fat is the primary energy source). But as soon as you rev up your motor—run, swim, dance aerobically, walk briskly—your muscles start to use up the stored carbohydrate to power your moving limbs. The harder or more intensely you exercise, the more carbohydrate (and proportionately less fat) you use for energy.

Also, during short bursts of activity, such as sprinting down the hallway to catch the elevator, climbing stairs, lifting weights, and other high-intensity exercises, your muscles can use only carbohydrates for energy. These activities are often called anaerobic exercises, referring to the use of glucose for energy without the use of incoming oxygen.

Clearly, your carbohydrate status—the amount of glycogen stored in the liver and muscles—dictates your performance. Staying competitive, whether it involves running a race or going through the daily grind in the workplace or at home, depends upon how well you keep your carbohydrate tanks filled. How much carbohydrate are you eating?

When you eat carbohydrate foods, like fruit, cereal, or bread, glucose goes into your bloodstream quickly, ready to provide immediate energy to the brain, muscles, or other body tissues demanding energy. If not immediately used for energy, glucose is stored away by the liver and muscles as glycogen. If you eat a low-carbohydrate diet, very little glycogen is stored in your body. The more carbohydrate you eat, the more glycogen you store, until your full capacity is achieved.

The amount of glycogen you store determines how long and at what level you can perform activities and continue to exercise. As you can see in the graph on page 41, the glycogen level is low with a daily diet low in carbohydrates. Exercising with this low level leads to early fatigue. In fact, on a low-carbohydrate diet (only about 40 percent of total calorie intake) your ability to last doing continuous exercise, like cycling, is about half that

CARB DIET LEVEL VS. MUSCLE GLYCOGEN LEVEL

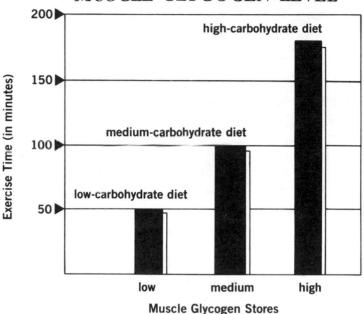

Glycogen stored in the muscles is the fuel that powers your exercise. The more carbohydrates in your diet, the greater your stores of glycogen—and the longer you can exercise without tiring.

SOURCE: Adapted from Bergstrom, et al., "Diet, Muscle Glycogen and Physical Performance." *Acta Physiol. Scand.* 71 (1967): 140.

compared with your ability on a high-carbohydrate diet (about 60 percent of total calorie intake).

Not only does the amount of carbohydrate in your diet affect an individual performance, such as a long exercise session, but on a daily basis your dietary carbohydrate dictates your day-to-day feelings of energy and fatigue. Are you powering through the day one step ahead, or does it seem the world is whizzing by while you're stuck in low gear?

You use large stores of glycogen in your muscles and liver every day, and even more on days with heavy activity (either continuous or short bursts of exercise). If you fail to eat enough

HOW MUSCLE GLYCOGEN LEVEL DECLINES WITH A LOW-CARB DIET

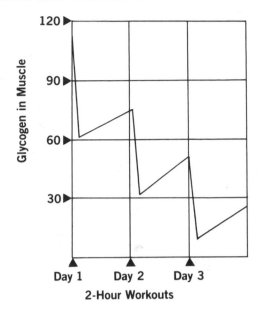

Without sufficient carbohydrates in the diet, after three consecutive days of two-hour workouts, nearly all muscle glycogen has been depleted.

SOURCE: Adapted from D. L. Costill et al., "Muscle Glycogen Utilization during Prolonged Exercise on Successive Days." *Journal of Applied Physiology* 31 (1971): 834–838.

carbohydrate to replenish your glycogen stores each day, the level of glycogen steadily declines, leaving you fatigued and unable to perform effectively.

You will especially notice the glycogen drain if you exercise routinely. After a few days of repeated workouts, you feel listless, tired, and uninterested in exercising. What used to be a manageable pace becomes fatiguing when you run low on glycogen. It is this day-by-day depletion of carbohydrate stores that I see most frequently in performing athletes and in individuals who put in exercise time, as well as active time at work or home, that requires bursts of activity.

Diane, a 37-year-old woman who works full-time and goes to

her health club four days a week, where she does either station-ary biking or aerobic dancing, found herself absolutely exhausted midway through her workouts. As Diane and I discussed her other activities (like climbing the stairs at her office at least seven or eight times a day) and her diet, the cause of her fatigue became apparent. She simply wasn't eating enough carbohy-drates day-in and day-out to keep her glycogen stores at a level needed to power both her exercise and work routine. Diet analysis showed that only 46 percent of her diet came from carbohydrates—far from the power-boosting optimum of 60 percent.

Avoiding daily fatigue and staying competitive requires eating a sufficient amount of carbohydrate on a daily basis. This is what the high-carbohydrate diet is all about—fueling yourself to meet your daily challenges. Later in this chapter, you'll find more on using carbohydrates to better your performance.

HOW TO EAT A HIGH-CARBOHYDRATE DIET

Staying energized with carbohydrates actually means eating carbo-rich foods in amounts you may view as excessive or "fat-tening." People often think of potatoes, pasta, and bread as "fat-tening" foods, when in fact these carbo-rich goodies energize more than they fatten. Surprisingly, your body is relatively ineffi-cient at converting excess dietary carbohydrate calories to body fat. Unlike the carbo-loaded bagel, the butter or cream cheese you may spread on it can easily be converted to body fat. If you eat more calories than you need to maintain your weight and support your exercise, you are better off if those excess calories come from carbohydrates. Here is how extra calories from fat and carbohydrates stack up:

□ If you eat 100 extra dietary fat calories, 97 end up as body fat and 3 calories are used for conversion to body fat.

□ If you eat 100 extra dietary carbohydrate calories, 77 end up as body fat and 23 calories are for conversion to body fat.

HOW MUCH CARBOHYDRATE DO YOU NEED?

Each of us has a different body, spends different amounts of time exercising, and faces different daily stresses and challenges.

Your need for carbohydrate, of course, depends upon your physical and mental demands. Allotting a percentage of your calorie intake to carbohydrates ensures that you meet those needs. The optimal level of carbohydrate calories depends upon how much you regularly tax your glycogen stores. Eating 58 to 70 percent of total calories from carbohydrates covers the needs of active people, including those who just tax their body stores of carbohydrate minimally and those who consistently work out several hours daily.

When you put this range of carbohydrate intake into perspective, you will soon achieve a diet higher in carbohydrate. Most of the athletes I work with, both casual and serious, come to me eating a diet that provides 45 to 55 percent of calories from carbs. When I show them their carbohydrate calorie percentage, most are shocked that they aren't reaching their goal of close to 60 percent. But few of them have any trouble making that goal once they learn simple ways to bump up their intake of carbohydrates, like switching from butter or margarine to fruit spread on breads, or choosing low-cal (low-fat) salad dressing.

In addition to the carbohydrate needed for performance, a certain amount of protein and fat is also necessary for health. The best way to look at the split between carbs, protein, and fat is to express each as a percentage of your total calorie intake. The optimal calorie breakdown that replenishes spent glycogen is 60 percent carbohydrate, 15 percent protein, and 25 percent fat.

Knowing what percentage of calories you presently get from carbohydrates is helpful, but not necessary. Through a computerized diet analysis, performed by a qualified dietitian/nutritionist, you can get the breakdown of calories from carbohydrate, fat, and protein in your diet. But you can get enough of this information for practical purposes by either adding up your daily total from reading food labels and using what I call "carb equivalents," or by following my simple guidelines on how to switch to a high-carb diet.

COUNTING CARBS

You can estimate the number of carbohydrate grams you need by converting your calorie intake into grams of carbohydrate.

Here is a simple method for making that conversion:

Step 1. Multiply the number of calories you take in daily (see below) by the percentage of carbohydrate calories you need (60 percent). This figure gives you the number of carbohydrate calories you need.

For active men, daily calorie needs range between 2,200 and 3,500 depending on exercise and other activities.

For active women, daily calorie needs range between 1,800 and 2,600 depending on exercise and other activities.

Example: 2,500 calories times 60 percent equals 1,500 calories needed from carbs.

Step 2. Compute the number of carbohydrate grams by dividing this number by 4 (carbohydrates provide 4 calories per gram) to get the number of carbohydrate grams needed.

Example: 1,500 calories divided by 4 calories/gram carbohydrate equals 375 grams of carbohydrate.

Calculate the number of carbohydrate grams you need and compare it with what you eat in a day. I usually have clients add up the amount of carbohydrate in the food they eat and compare this with their carbo goal of 60 percent. Using Tables 2-1 and 2-3 and the carbohydrate information on food labels, you can easily see if you are close to your mark.

Check labels on packaged foods like cereals, TV dinners, canned soups, and snack foods. Listed on the nutrition panel is the number of carbohydrate grams. Use this value to add up your daily carb total, paying attention to how many servings you will have. Here is a typical nutrition panel:

> *Macaroni and Cheese*
> *Nutrition information*
> *Serving: 1 cup*
> *Calories: 260*
> *Protein: 9 grams*
> *Carbohydrate: 26 grams*
> *Fat: 13 grams*

DON'T BE TAKEN FOR A FAT RIDE

You can also use the food label information to compute the percentage of carbohydrate calories you get when you eat what's

Table 2-1 CONVENIENT HIGH-CARBOHYDRATE FOODS

Food	Portion	Calories	Carbohydrate (g)	Calories from Carbohydrate (%)
Bagel	1	160	31	78
Banana	1 large	120	30	95
Bread, wheat or white	2 slices	160	30	75
Bread sticks	4	154	30	78
Cereal, ready-to-eat, flake-type	1 cup	110	25	90
Corn on the cob	1 ear	120	29	95
Crackers, low-fat	½ large	80	20	100
Dried fruit (raisins, apricots)	½ cup	225	50	89
Fruit juice	1 cup	120	30	100
Kidney beans, canned	1 cup	186	35	75
Pancakes	3 (4 in.)	260	51	78
Popcorn, plain	4 cups	92	18	78
Potato, baked	1 large	220	51	93
Pretzels, low-salt	2 oz.	222	43	77
Rice cakes	5	200	40	80

SOURCE: Adapted from J. A. T. Pennington, *Bowes and Church's Food Values of Portions Commonly Used*, 15th ed. (Philadelphia: J. B. Lippincott, 1989).

in the box. This formula helps you to identify whether a food is high-carb or high-fat.

Step 1. Multiply the grams of carbohydrate given on the label by 4. This gives you carbohydrate calories.

Step 2. Compare the number of carbohydrate calories to the total number of calories per serving of the packaged food to get a percentage of carbohydrate calories.

Example: For packaged macaroni and cheese: 26 grams of carbohydrate times 4 calories/gram carbohydrate equals 104 calories; 104 calories of carbohydrate in 260 calories per serving equals 40 percent.

Macaroni and cheese is only 40 percent carbohydrate—not very high for a pasta dish and nowhere near our 60 percent goal!

Table 2-2 *"HIGH-CARB" FOODS WITH HIDDEN FAT*

Although these foods are commonly seen as good carbohydrate sources, they actually pack a dose of fat.

Food	Calories from Fat (%)
Bran muffin, bakery type	41
Burrito, packaged	45
Carrot cake	38
Cheese pizza, frozen	44
Cookies	35–55
Corn chips	51
Croissant	50
Doughnut, cake type	47
Pasta with cream sauce	40
Popcorn, microwave, butter flavor	54
Potato chips	60
Waffles	44

SOURCE: Adapted from J. A. T. Pennington, *Bowes and Church's Food Values of Portions Commonly Used,* 15th ed. (Philadelphia: J. B. Lippincott, 1989).

(In chapter 4, you calculate fat calories in packaged foods.)

It is surprising to discover that many supposedly high-carbohydrate foods are actually high-fat foods. I find that many people turn to these foods, wanting to believe they are loading up on carbs. Look at Table 2-2 for a list of foods commonly mistaken as high-carb, to see if you're being taken for a fat ride.

Besides using a food label to tally your carbo score, you should also use what I call the "carb equivalents," listed in Table 2-3. Because not all the food we eat (fruits and vegetables, for example) is conveniently labeled, I use the carb equivalents to estimate their carbohydrate content.

Try adding up your daily carbohydrate intake once in the beginning when you are making the switch from your present diet, and again when you feel comfortable with the changes you have made in your eating style. Table 2-4 shows one day's diet record of a client who felt she was too busy to stop for lunch. Cathy, an advertising executive, ended up snacking her way to a listless low-carbohydrate diet. After learning how to add up carbohydrates, she quickly became wary of her high-fat snacking habits and made the healthful switch you see.

It is not necessary to add up your carbohydrate score daily, but do so if you feel better about your diet by keeping close tabs. In Part 2, I show you how to use carb equivalents when you're dining out, traveling, or munching from the vending machine at work. Using these numbers can keep you on the high-performance track.

SIMPLIFY HIGH-CARBO EATING

When starting people off on the high-performance, high-carbohydrate diet, I first get them practicing substitutions—replacing foods that are low in carbohydrate and high in fat with foods that give plenty of energizing carbs. As I mentioned before, your diet is a balance of foods that provide the nourishment you need to perform. Beyond carbohydrates, you need protein, vitamins, minerals, and even some fat to perform optimally. In chapters 3, 4, and 5, I cover the role of these nutrients in more detail. But right now it's important to realize how essential it is to consume sufficient carbohydrates for stamina and performance.

Table 2-3 *CARB EQUIVALENTS*

The following four categories of foods are the major carbohydrate sources in your diet. Write down what you eat for one day, then tally up your carbohydrate score by adding the number of grams for each serving of carbohydrate food you ate.

Food	Portion
Starch: Bread, Cereals, Crackers, Grains	
(15 g carbohydrate/serving)	
Bagel	½
Bread	1 slice
Bread sticks	2
Cereals, bran (such as All Bran)	½ cup
Cereals, cooked	½ cup
Cereals, ready-to-eat	¾ cup
Corn	½ cup; one 6 in. ear
Crackers, soda, whole wheat, no added fat	¾ oz.
Kidney beans	⅓ cup
Lentils	⅓ cup
Lima beans	½ cup
Pasta, cooked	½ cup
Pita bread	½
Popcorn	3 cups
Potato, baked	1 small
Potato, mashed	½ cup
Pretzels	¾ oz.
Rice	⅓ cup
Tortilla	1 (6 in.)
White beans	⅓ cup
Winter squash	¾ cup
Yam, sweet potato	⅓ cup
Fruit and Fruit Juice (15 g carbohydrate/serving)	
Apple	1 small

(continued)

Table 2-3—*Continued*

Food	Portion
Fruit and Fruit Juice (15 g carbohydrate/serving)	
Applesauce	½ cup
Banana	½
Cantaloupe	⅓
Dried fruit	¼ cup
Fruit juice	½ cup
Orange	1 small
Pineapple	¾ cup
Strawberries, whole	1¼ cup
Vegetable and Vegetable Juice (5 g carbohydrate/serving)	
Beans, green	½ cup cooked; 1 cup raw
Beets	½ cup cooked; 1 cup raw
Broccoli	½ cup cooked; 1 cup raw
Cabbage	½ cup cooked; 1 cup raw
Cauliflower	½ cup cooked; 1 cup raw
Onions	½ cup cooked; 1 cup raw
Peppers	½ cup cooked; 1 cup raw
Spinach	½ cup cooked; 1 cup raw
Summer squash	½ cup cooked; 1 cup raw
Tomato	½ cup cooked or juice; 1 cup raw
Water chestnuts	½ cup cooked; 1 cup raw
Milk and Milk Products (12 g carbohydrate/serving)	
Low-fat, 1%, or skim milk	1 cup
Low-fat buttermilk	1 cup
Low-fat/nonfat plain yogurt	8 oz.

As you begin to change your eating style, view your diet as a series of options—each meal and snack you select is a choice you make toward improving your performance. Instead of attempting to alter your entire diet overnight, look at the individual food choices and how each can be changed to better your performance and stamina. Don't think of eating for better performance as a chore, but as a natural progression in your eating style based on the successes you have as a result of the changes in your diet.

Table 2-4 *SCHEDULE FOR A BUSY EXECUTIVE*

Here's a sample of one woman's transformation from a high-fat, low-energy diet to high-performance eating.

Before	After
7:30—Breakfast	
2 muffins (bakery type)	*Homemade blender drink:*
Coffee with cream	½ cup nonfat yogurt
	1 banana
	½ cup orange juice
12:00—Lunch	
Vending machine snack:	*Take-out lunch:*
Packaged cheese spread and	Turkey sandwich
crackers	Carrot sticks
	Peach
2:00—Lunch in Office	
Pastrami deli sandwich	—
Diet soda	
4:00—Snack at Desk	
Handful of snack crackers	RyKrisp
	1 can V-8 juice
7:00—While Making Dinner	
1 glass wine	1 glass wine
"Nibbles" of cheese (2 oz.)	Raw vegetables dipped in yogurt and herbs
7:30—Dinner	
TV dinner, lite type	Broiled fish with lemon/garlic sauce
Tossed green salad with dressing	Tossed green salad with low-cal dressing
Dinner roll with 1 tsp. margarine	
10:30—TV Snack	
4 chocolate cookies	3 cups popcorn
1 glass low-fat milk	1 glass skim milk
Analysis	
Total calories: 1,980	Total calories: 1,970
31% carbohydrate	61% carbohydrate
48% fat	17% fat

In Table 2-5 I provide you with lists of alternatives to high-fat, low-nutrition foods. Use these, along with the lists in "Top Complex-Carbohydrate Foods" on page 38, to start revamping your daily food selections.

Table 2-5 *BOOST YOUR DAILY CARBOHYDRATE INTAKE*

Switch to these easy alternatives to standard high-fat snacks.

Instead of . . .	Choose . . .
Chocolate bar	Fruit, fruit juice, moderate amounts of hard candy
Doughnuts, pastries	Bran or corn muffins (watch for fat content), bagels
Ice cream	Fruit ice, sherbet, ice milk, fruit bars, frozen yogurt
Milkshakes	Skim milk blenderized with bananas or other fruit, chocolate syrup, and ice
Nuts	Dried fruit or power fruit mix
Potato or corn chips	Pretzels, whole-grain crackers, soda crackers, rice cakes
Shortbread or cream-filled cookies	Vanilla wafers, gingersnaps, animal crackers, fig bars, graham crackers
Snack crackers	Popcorn, whole-grain crackers

For most active people, it's often easier to compare what you presently eat to planned menus that are "just what the doctor ordered." I give meal plans to clients who eat out often and find it tricky to evaluate carbs and fats in foods listed on restaurant menus. I recently met a financial analyst who traveled and ate out often. He found that a list of complete, high-carbohydrate meals was more useful than a list of food substitutions.

Table 2-6 *MEAL MAKEOVERS*

Move to high-performance carbohydrates from high-fat eating.

High-Fat (Before)	High-Carbohydrate (After)
Breakfast	
At fast-food restaurant	
1 croissant breakfast sandwich	2 bagels and fruit spread
6 ounces orange juice	1 cup low-fat yogurt with ¾ cup strawberries
Coffee with cream	Coffee with low-fat milk
Lunch	
At restaurant	
2 cups pasta with seafood and cream sauce	2 cups bean chili
Tossed green salad with house dressing	Salad with vinegar or lemon juice dressing
1 slice French bread with butter	2 slices French bread
	¾ cup fruit sorbet
Dinner	
Take-out	
2 egg rolls	Stir-fry vegetables
1 cup fried rice	1 cup steamed rice
1 cup chow mein	1 cup beef and broccoli stir-fry
1 ice cream cone	5 fig bars
Analysis	
Total calories: 2,420	Total calories: 2,220
42% carbohydrate	60% carbohydrate
40% fat	24% fat

If you eat organized meals—that is, breakfast, lunch, and dinner—compare what you eat with the before and after meals listed in Table 2-6. Later, I'll cover more performance meals, as well as how to manage sporadic eating, missing meals, and grazing.

STAY COMPETITIVE WITH CARBOHYDRATES: FOR ATHLETES AT ANY AGE

We all know that carbohydrates are vital for stamina and performance. Carbohydrates also keep you running with the pack, and even ahead of it, if you know how to harness the miracle of carbohydrates. Now here is my guide to using carbs so you can boost your stamina, ward off fatigue, and stay competitive throughout your race, whether it's a true competition or a relaxing weekend jog.

I'll cover the steps you need to take before your event from several days to minutes before start time. Also, I'll show you what's best to eat during competition for top-notch performance.

FILLING YOUR TANKS: CARBO-LOADING

You know that the amount of glycogen you have stored in your muscles and liver determines the length and quality of your exercise performance. So it follows that low glycogen stores will force you to reduce your pace, or stop altogether, as you fatigue in any exercise you do lasting 60 to 90 minutes or more.

Boosting your glycogen stores with a high-carb diet means more power longer. Storing glycogen the right way before your competition will prevent you from "hitting the wall," a term endurance athletes use to describe the heavy, leadlike feeling your legs have when glycogen runs out—the feeling that you can't take another step. Low glycogen forces your body to slow down automatically and switch to using more body fat for energy.

Filling your glycogen tanks before a race is simple—but it must be done the right way.

1. Eat lots of carbohydrates.

2. Give your muscles a bit of rest to allow carbohydrate stores to top off.

This is what I call "loaf loading," a modification of the classic carbohydrate-loading scheme developed in the 1970s (see Table 2-7). The classic scheme involves extremes in training and diet that leave athletes feeling tired and sluggish, and it may impair their performance. The new loaf-loading approach, developed by W. Mike Sherman, Ph.D., and Dave Costill, Ph.D., is a safer, more effective way to raise body glycogen stores for long exercise.

Both procedures increase glycogen stores to their maximum, but the modified plan allows athletes to do so without risk. Weight loss, weakness, even heart-rhythm problems can occur in athletes who use the classic method. Furthermore, requiring a few days on a low-carbohydrate diet makes training next to impossible. On a first-hand basis, I found the classic carbo-loading routine both physically and mentally fatiguing.

Moreover, since water is normally stored in the muscles with glycogen, sudden weight gain (five to ten pounds) may occur in athletes who follow the classic carbo-loading method, causing obvious performance problems. In the loaf-loading scheme, water weight gain is spread over several days and is not as great as in the classic carbo-loading routine, since athletes don't exhaust glycogen stores completely.

While the exact reason that muscles pack away extra carbohydrate for energy is not known, researchers find that resting the muscles allows them to soak up more carbohydrate. Among athletes who don't allow their muscles adequate time for recovery, performance often suffers.

A number of the athletes I work with fight this rest issue. It took me the better part of one race season to convince Alan, a hard-driving, 46-year-old agricultural chemist, to cut back on training a few days before entering a biathlon (bike/run race). He felt a 30-mile ride the day before a race would get him warmed up for it, but the ride was actually depleting his glycogen stores. I made a bet with Alan that he would feel stronger during his race if he rested the day before. He tried it, and sure enough, he had his best race ever, despite the fact that the chain fell off his bike midway through his ride! Since it takes 24 to 48 hours to recover spent glycogen stores fully, it is better to rest or exercise *very lightly* the day before an endurance race.

I like to think of carbo-loading as though you were storing away slices of bread in your body for your muscles to eat during exercise. This system actually buys you time—you can exercise about 60 minutes longer, or better withstand more high-intensity

Table 2-7 *CARBOHYDRATE-LOADING SCHEMES*

Time before Event	Loaf-Loading Method		Classical Method	
	Training	Diet	Training	Diet
6 days	90 min. (hard intensity)	55–60% carbs (typical training diet)	90–120 min. (hard intensity)	50% carbs
5 days	40–60 min. (moderate)	55–60% carbs	40–60 min. (moderate)	Low-carb diet (10% carbs)
4 days	30–40 min. (moderate)	60–70% carbs	40–60 min. (moderate)	Low-carb diet
3 days	20–30 min. (moderate)	70% carbs	40–60 min. (moderate)	Low-carb diet
2 days	20 min. (mild-loaf part)	70% carbs	30–40 min. (moderate)	High-carb diet (90% carbs)
1 day	Rest	70% carbs	Rest	High-carb diet
Event	—	—	—	—

activity like weight lifting or sprinting. Of course, your muscles store more glycogen when you are in good shape than when you are not. So if you are well trained, even if you don't carbo load, your muscles already have a fair amount of stored carbohydrate, and carbo-loading boosts this level. On the other hand, if you are out of shape, carbo-loading won't do much for your glycogen stores and performance.

Here's a comparison of a man's carbohydrate energy stores before and after carbo-loading:
1. Well-trained athlete "unloaded"—1,700 calories of stored energy (equivalent to 28 slices of bread).
2. Well-trained athlete "loaded"—2,300 calories of stored energy (equivalent to 38 slices of bread).

CARBO-LOADING HOW-TO's

If you follow the time course given in Table 2-7 and use what you now know about carbohydrate-rich foods, carbo-loading should be a cinch and shouldn't interfere with your day-to-day routine. Because you are already eating a diet that is at least 60 percent carbohydrate calories, you need to modify your diet only slightly two days before competition. During these days, you need to eat approximately 70 percent of your calories as carbohydrate. This means cutting back a bit on fat and adding more complex-carbo foods such as pasta, potatoes, cereals, and breads.

Practically speaking, those extra carbohydrates do not include ice cream, chocolate, high-fat cheeses, fatty snack crackers, chips, or alcohol. During my final days before a competition, I try to eat more carbs by switching to fruits for dessert even though I love ice cream, sticking to my usual breakfast of whole-grain cereal with skim milk, and avoiding any dishes that include heavy cream sauces. The meal suggestions in "The Day before the Race: A High-Carbo Menu" on page 60 contain approximately 70 percent of total calories as carbohydrate. Remember, the idea during these few days is to increase carbohydrate calories, not to "pig out" and gain weight. You should feel well rested and light on your feet after "carbing up," not sluggish and tired.

Many people tell me they don't want the hassle of changing

Table 2-8 *CARB-LOADING FOOD AND DRINK*

You can use these high-carbohydrate foods and liquid supplements for easy loading.

Item	Portion	Calories	Carbohydrate (g)	Calories from Carbohydrate (%)
Foods				
Bagels	2	320	62	78
Banana	1 large	120	30	95
Bread, white or wheat	4 slices	320	60	75
Pancakes	3 (4 in.)	260	51	78
Pasta, cooked	2 cups	320	67	84
Popcorn	6 cups	138	28	81
Potato, baked	1 large	220	51	93
Rice, brown, cooked	1 cup	232	50	86
Liquids (made to manufacturer's directions)				
Carbo Energizer	8 oz.	237	59	100
Carbofuel	8 oz.	334	80	100
Carboplex	8 oz.	218	54	100
Exceed High Carbohydrate Source	8 oz.	235	59	100
GatorLode	8 oz.	187	47	100
Paragon Fast Recovery	8 oz.	240	60	100
Ultra Fuel	8 oz.	200	50	100

SOURCE: Food values adapted from J. A. T. Pennington, *Bowes and Church's Food Values of Portions Commonly Used*, 15th ed. (Philadelphia: J. B. Lippincott, 1989).

NOTE: Data for liquids derived from product labels.

the kinds of food they eat to make sure they get enough carbs. "Couldn't I just drink some glycogen!?!" asked 25-year-old Mark, who didn't cook for himself. (Mark's day was spent either at work or working out, and he preferred to eat ready-made food.) I told him that he couldn't actually drink glycogen, but he could use carbohydrate supplements, such as Exceed High Carbohydrate Source and GatorLode. When dissolved in water, they become concentrated carbohydrate drinks that can substitute for potatoes and pasta. These drinks are easy to use, and for people like Mark who don't want to cook, such carb supplements are a convenient alternative. Look for prepackaged carbo supplements that are fortified with B vitamins, essential for releasing the energy you've packed away. Compared with complex-carbohydrate foods (bread, cereals, potatoes), canned carbo sources are much more expensive, but they contribute equally to glycogen storage.

THE DAY BEFORE COMPETITION: STICK TO BASICS

I have seen many athletes run into problems during a race because of what they ate or didn't eat (not eating enough the day before and running out of energy during the race is typical). Also, an athlete might eat an unusual food for the first time (a new power supplement or drink) that ends up causing stomach problems on race morning.

Some athletes think that if they eat only a little bit, or even go without food altogether the day before a race, they will feel light on their feet. They couldn't be more wrong! Skimping on food the day before only saps those precious glycogen stores that were built up so carefully. In fact, in less than 24 hours of not eating, you can drain your liver glycogen stores completely, without any exercise at all. This leaves your brain short on fuel and can result in a crash due to delirium early in your race.

Even skipping dinner the night before cuts into your glycogen stores by race time the next morning. Your body uses carbs even while you sleep, so cutting back on food the day before means digging deeper into your carbo reserves. A top woman triathlete I worked with couldn't believe how much better she felt during her races after she took my suggestion to eat dinner the night

THE DAY BEFORE THE RACE: A HIGH-CARBO MENU

Breakfast

1½ cups whole-grain cereal (NutriGrain, oatmeal, 9-grain, or the like)

1 cup skim milk

2 bagels with 2 tablespoons fruit spread

1 orange

1 banana

Snack

3½ ounces dried fruit (peaches and apricots mixed)

Lunch

2 sandwiches: 4 slices whole-wheat bread, water-packed tuna mixed with 2 tablespoons reduced-calorie mayonnaise or low-fat yogurt (4 ounces total)

2 raw carrots

½ cantaloupe

2 rice cakes

½ cup raisins

Snack

1 apple

1 cup nonfat fruit-flavored yogurt

Dinner

2 cups cooked brown rice topped with 1½ cups stir-fry vegetables (broccoli, onions, bok choy) and 4 ounces tofu or 3 ounces cooked chicken

2 cups green salad (leaf lettuce) with 2 tablespoons yogurt-based dressing

1 cup frozen yogurt topped with ¾ cup fresh fruit (strawberries, melon, nectarines)

Analysis

Total calories: 3,100. Distribution: 70 percent carbohydrate, 15 percent protein, 15 percent fat.

before. Because she was worried about feeling sluggish, she tried a light dinner (cereal and fruit) at first. Soon she found that eating a high-complex-carbohydrate dinner (her favorite was pizza crust and cranberry juice!) worked very well.

It's very important to stay away from unfamiliar food the night before the race. Eating ethnic food you don't ordinarily eat, such as Mexican or Chinese, is a common mistake. The spices and other unfamiliar ingredients may not sit well with you, particularly if you suffer from prerace nerves. This type of problem commonly occurs when athletes travel to distant races and eat what sounds good rather than what is sensible.

Also, many competitors load up on salads and other fibrous foods the day before the race in an effort to stuff carbohydrates. Unfortunately, the consequence for some is "runner's trots," frequent bowel movements during competition. If anything, I suggest you moderate your fiber intake, stick to amounts you are used to, and avoid fiber supplements on the day before you race. So, if your breakfast is usually bran cereal, eat an extra piece of fruit or a bagel for added carbohydrate rather than two bowls of bran cereal.

I always eat before I race. But what I eat depends upon how

THE NIGHT BEFORE THE RACE: A HIGH-CARBO DINNER

Sample Menu

- 2 baked potatoes topped with 1 cup steamed broccoli and ⅓ cup low-fat cheddar cheese or mozzarella cheese
- 2 whole-wheat or white dinner rolls with fruit spread
- 1 glass skim milk or iced herb tea (decaffeinated)
- 1 cup low-fat frozen yogurt topped with ½ cup fresh fruit

Analysis

Total calories: 1,340 (81 percent from carbohydrate)

I expect my body to perform. And I urge all athletes to consider what they are about to put their bodies through and eat accordingly.

Eating before you exercise can help or harm your performance, so choose carefully when and what you eat. The few hours before you compete can be nerve-racking, very different from the calm of a training day. Thus, the nourishment you give your body before exercise should be a performance booster, but not anything to unsettle your stomach. Here are the basics of prerace eating.

First, after a night's sleep, you have been without food for 12 to 15 hours, and you need something to keep your energy level up. If you plan to exercise without eating, remember that doing so will sap your glycogen stores more rapidly and you will run out of energy. When you train in the morning, most likely you don't eat anything before and do just fine. But on race day, timing is usually different and you end up going for a longer period without food. You need a source of carbohydrate to keep your blood sugar level normal and to prevent feelings of hunger and weakness.

Second, a race or athletic event that lasts longer than about 90 minutes requires more carbohydrate than you normally have stored in your muscles and liver as glycogen. Eating some carbohydrate a number of hours before competing will top off glycogen stores. Also, eating a good dose of carbohydrate foods before you compete in a longer event can actually boost your performance beyond what you can do after eating just a small meal or nothing at all. This advice is contrary to that given by nutritionists in the past. Typically, I advise athletes to eat a light meal (at least 500 calories, mostly carbs) about three hours before exercise to avoid stomach upset. New research suggests that more carbs may be even better for a long run.

Studies carried out by W. Mike Sherman, Ph.D., at Ohio State University showed that eating a large amount of carbohydrate (say 1,400 calories, the amount in 23 slices of bread) three hours before exercise enabled cyclists to pedal 20 percent longer than cyclists who ate nothing before they rode. This large dose of carbohydrate, which was taken as a liquid carbohydrate drink such as Exceed High Carbohydrate Source, supplied the working muscles with precious carbohydrate energy so that exercise could continue.

I recommend eating or drinking carbohydrates as close as one hour before exercise. In the past, athletes have avoided eating carbohydrates one hour before exercise on the advice of nutritionists. This was done to prevent undesirable changes in blood sugar levels due to the release of insulin, a hormone needed to process carbohydrate. A drop in blood sugar before the start of exercise could mean a more rapid use of glycogen stores. However, new research shows this drop in blood sugar is transient and does not adversely affect performance.

When athletes were fed 300 calories of carbohydrate one hour before a cycling test, blood sugar levels dropped at the start of exercise, but were soon normalized. These athletes went on to cycle faster than athletes who didn't receive a carbo snack right before exercise. This research suggests that a pre-exercise snack provides the added sugar energy needed for high-intensity exercise, such as a finishing kick at the end of a run.

This is information you can and should use for prerace eating strategies in your training. If you improve your performance with better prerace eating, then faster training will lead to faster racing. Experiment first with meal timing. If you race, plan to eat a meal one to four hours before exercise. Don't worry about exercising with food in your stomach, since athletes seem to process a high-carbohydrate meal more rapidly than untrained individuals do.

When considering what to eat, stick to high-carbohydrate foods or drinks. Fats and protein are digested more slowly and are not the limiting energy factor during exercise. Good prerace foods are low-fiber cereals, breads, low-fat muffins, bagels, or fruit.

How much to eat depends upon your body size and how long you will be exercising. For short events, you are better off eating between 300 and 600 calories, mostly from carbohydrates. But for longer races, you will need more calories. Researchers at Ohio State fed athletes about 9 calories per pound of body weight (about 1,400 calories for a 155-pound athlete). If you are eating one hour before exercise, however, you will want to cut this back to about 2 calories per pound of body weight, or about 310 calories.

You will need to calibrate yourself on meal size, since the larger the meal, the greater the chances of stomach upset. Also, keep in mind that prerace nerves may also make food more difficult to tolerate. Some athletes find solid foods are more difficult to handle as a prerace meal than liquid foods. Since liquids empty from the stomach quickly and leave little residue in the intestines which may cause discomfort while exercising, I often recommend liquid carbohydrate supplements as a prerace meal.

If you're looking for more than carbohydrate for a prerace meal, liquid-food products, such as Nutrament or Exceed Sports Nutritional Supplement, are complete meals which also work well as pre-exercise meals. Be sure to check the label on packaged carbohydrate products, since some may be high in fat and/or protein. Table 2-9 lists some products for you to compare. A word of caution, however: Taste them before race day so there are no unpleasant surprises.

I also recommend "energy bars" as a good prerace meal. Many of these products are high in carbohydrate and low in fat, taste good, and transport well, making them excellent prerace meals if you have to travel to the race. Check Table 2-10 for energy bar comparisons. As with the liquid products, you should try them before race day so you are familiar with their taste.

The key to racing success lies in your training. Take time now to figure your perfect prerace meal, and don't change anything on race day unless you have good reason to do so. "Prerace Menus" on page 67 lists my suggestions for prerace meals for various race-start times.

FUELING DURING EXERCISE

I have had disappointing performances of my own, of course; not for lack of training or mental readiness, but mostly for lack of a good eating plan. My own experiences, along with results from research, have helped me formulate refueling plans for athletes participating in events lasting anywhere from 1 to 20 hours! Together, we can develop a refueling plan that will work for you.

Table 2-9 *LIQUID PRERACE MEALS*

These easy-to-stomach meals are excellent choices prior to a race (1 to 3 hours before).

Product	Calories	Calories from Carbohydrate (%)
Ensure Plus (Ross Lab)	355	53
Exceed Sports Nutritional Supplement (Ross Lab; specifically designed for prerace use)	360	60
Gator Pro (Quaker Oats)	360	64
Go! (Nutri-Products)	190	57
Sego Liquid diet meal (Pet)	225	60
Sustical (Mead Johnson)	240	55

NOTE: Data derived from product labels.

Table 2-10 *"ENERGY" BARS: A PRERACE CONVENIENCE*

Product	Calories	Calories from Carbohydrate (%)
Exceed Sports Bar	280	76
FinHalsa	170	64
Meal-on-the-Go	290	61
Nu-Treat	231	70
Pemmican Fruit'n Nut	420	56
Power Bar	225	71

NOTE: Data derived from product labels.

POWER FOODS: THE FACTS

Your decision to eat during exercise should be based upon how long you plan to be performing, how intensely you intend to exercise, and your individual experience with eating while exercising. As with prerace eating, you are in continuing need of carbohydrates during long-term exercise—your muscles will perform better if well fed with carbs.

As you exercise, your muscles use up stored carbohydrates and become thirsty for a replenishing supply of sugar from the blood. It is the role of your liver to supply this sugar, but it, too, is running out of carbohydrates. This drying up of body carbohydrates, particularly when blood sugar levels drop, brings on the "bonk," a feeling of light-headedness and weakness. Drinking a sport drink or eating a carbohydrate food will give your muscles and brain this crucial supply of carbohydrates to delay inevitable fatigue.

Along with carbohydrates, your body is in need of thirst-quenching fluids to replace large quantities lost due to heavy sweating. I cover fluid replacement strategies in chapter 1, along with choosing the "right" sport drink. What you should understand now is the importance of taking a carbohydrate source during exercise lasting over one hour, and how carbohydrate is needed to ward off fatigue.

Whether you choose a solid food, such as a banana, or a sport drink, try to get about 100 to 150 calories for every half hour of exercise. The right amount for you depends upon your body size and how intensely you exercise. Choosing solid food over a liquid source of carbohydrate depends upon your preference. I personally use both solid and liquid carbohydrates during a long stretch of exercise. Many athletes want solid foods to help take away that hollow, hungry feeling that sport drinks don't alleviate.

You should start to eat soon after you begin to exercise, if you know you will be going for at least 60 to 90 minutes. Some athletes need to eat only if they exercise for two hours or more. Decide this on the basis of your own experience. In any case, don't wait until you are light-headed and weak before you eat. Replenishing carbohydrates throughout exercise will ensure better performance. If you put off eating until near the end of your race, a jolt of carbohydrates will still help your perfor-

PRERACE MENUS

Different race times demand different meal plans. Here are suggestions based on the needs of a 140- to 160-pound person for three start times. Tailor your prerace eating to your body weight and food likes.

7:30 A.M. Race Start

Resist skipping your pre-exercise meal at this early hour. Eat a light meal (300 to 600 calories) one to two hours before start time.

- 3 slices dry toast
- 1 banana or 1 to 2 cans Exceed Nutritional Supplement

11:30 A.M. Race Start

With a late-morning start, plan to eat a good-sized meal (about 1,100 calories) at 7:00 or 8:00 A.M.

- 2 cups whole-grain flake cereal
- 1 cup skim milk
- 2 bagels with 2 tablespoons fruit spread
- 2 pieces of fruit: peach, pear
- 1 large blueberry muffin

6:00 P.M. Race Start

An end-of-the-day race should be run on a low-fat breakfast and lunch and an early-afternoon high-carb snack.

Breakfast: about 720 calories

- 4 slices French toast with syrup
- 12 ounces V-8 juice
- 8 ounces low-fat milk
- 1 cup fresh fruit compote

Lunch: about 850 calories

- 1 large baked potato topped with ½ cup plain yogurt, steamed broccoli, and 2 ounces cheddar cheese
- 1 thick slice whole-grain bread
- 8 ounces orange juice
- 2 medium-size apples

Snack (3:00 P.M.): about 430 calories

- 2 cups carbohydrate supplement drink *or*
- 6 fig bars *and*
- 8 ounces apple juice

mance, since carbs are rapidly absorbed and quickly sent out to the bloodstream, energizing your carbo-thirsty muscles.

Choose your race food carefully. Test your racing foods and replacement schedule during training: Don't risk potential stomach problems from a new food during a race. Avoid foods high in fat or protein—these two nutrients will do nothing for you during a race except retard performance. I list some excellent race foods in Table 2-11. Using these, along with the refueling guidelines in chapter 1, will help you perform your best.

RECOVERY EATING: THE RIGHT WAY TO RECHARGE AFTER EXERCISE OR HARD WORK

When you push for your best performance—a hard morning run out on the roads or a demanding day at the office—you are draining valuable energy stores. If you recharge the right way, you will be ready for yet another demanding performance. My plan for a quick rebound includes eating the right foods, timing your meals wisely, and rehydrating adequately. Follow my guidelines to ensure speedy recovery after you've sapped your energy.

Recovery measures after vigorous exercise or after a ten-hour workday have much in common. Yet there are some different steps to take in each case. First I'll show a recovery strategy after a hard workout, then I'll show how to bounce back the next day after a traumatic day at the office.

AFTER EXERCISE

Bicycling, running, or brisk walking for long stretches of time deplete both your glycogen stores and vital body water lost as sweat. It takes anywhere from 24 to 48 hours for full recovery, provided you are eating a high-carbohydrate diet and consuming plenty of fluids. An average man who weighs 160 pounds, for instance, needs about 2,400 carbohydrate calories to fill up his glycogen tanks. This represents 600 grams of carbohydrate, the amount found in 40 slices of bread. Eating this large amount of carbohydrate is usually manageable over a 1½- to 3-day period, but if you expect to race or even work out within 24 to 48 hours of your last exercise bout, rapid replacement of glycogen stores is crucial. Follow my six proven steps for rapid recovery.

Table 2-11 *RACE FOODS*

Here's a list of easy-to-take-along high-carb foods to eat during racing or training. Use 100 calories every 30 minutes as a starting point, and tailor your race-day eating to your needs.

Food	Portion	Calories
Apple	1	80
Apricots, dried	¼ cup	80
Bagel	1	160
Banana	1	120
Bread	1 slice	80
Dates	5	125
Fig bars	2	100
Figs	3	120
Fruit leather	1 oz.	100
Gingersnaps	3	90
Grapes	1 cup	60
Melon pieces	1 cup	55
Peach, fresh	1	40
Peaches, dried	¼ cup	96
Pear, fresh	1	90
Pears, dried	¼ cup	115
Potato, baked	1 medium	140
Prunes	¼ cup	95
Raisin-filled biscuits	1	50
Raisins	¼ cup	110
Rice, sweetened (with 1 tsp. sugar)	½ cup	95
Vanilla wafers	5	90

SOURCE: Adapted from J. A. T. Pennington, *Bowes and Church's Food Values of Portions Commonly Used,* 15th ed. (Philadelphia: J. B. Lippincott, 1989).

1. Eat carbohydrate within one hour after exercise. Research studies show that you can expect to achieve full recovery of glycogen stores only if you begin carbohydrate reloading almost immediately after exercise.

A recent study showed that cyclists who consumed carbohydrates immediately after exercise replaced depleted muscle glycogen 50 percent faster than cyclists who delayed carbohydrate consumption for two hours. And when muscle glycogen levels were measured again later, the cyclists who received the delayed feeding still had not resynthesized as much glycogen as subjects who had eaten the same dose of carbohydrates immediately.

Chowing down soon after a draining workout or race may not be appealing, particularly since your appetite might be less than hearty after hard exercise. Waiting an hour before you eat won't hurt, but postponing a carbo-rich meal two to four hours will hinder your short-term recovery.

2. Eat enough carbohydrate. Nibbling on bread after exercise just won't do the job—you really have to make an effort to eat more carbo-rich foods after exercise than you would normally opt for. You must consume one to two carbohydrate calories for each pound of body weight every two hours to bring glycogen stores back up at an optimal rate. For example, for a 120-pound person, this translates to four slices of bread every two hours (or one bagel and two apples, or one orange and nine cups of air-popped popcorn).

Before you overdose on popcorn and bread, however, remember that eating more carbohydrates than you need won't speed your glycogen recovery rate. Studies have shown that even doubling this carbohydrate dosage doesn't help you recover lost glycogen any faster.

3. Eat small meals or snacks. You can also maximize glycogen storage by eating small or more frequent carbohydrate meals during the hours after exercise instead of eating one or two large meals. Studies performed on laboratory animals suggest that "grazing" on carbohydrates provides a steady supply of glucose to recovering muscles. Also, small meals or snacks are better tolerated, since your appetite may be touchy soon after exercise.

Try a liquid carbohydrate source to augment carbohydrate intake if you can't quite stomach any solid food immediately after exercise. Most liquid carbohydrate sources consist of complex carbohydrates, similar to starch. Dissolved in water, these products contain about twice the carbohydrate concentration of fruit juice and almost four times the carbohydrate concentration of most sport drinks. Use carbohydrate supplements during the hours after exercise, but not as a complete substitute for carbohydrate foods, which provide vitamins, minerals, and fiber needed for overall health and performance.

4. Choose your carbohydrates wisely. Your choice of carbohydrates influences how quickly you recover lost glycogen. You have two options: glucose and fructose, both of which are monosaccharides. Glucose is found in most carbohydrate food sources—breads, potatoes, and vegetables, for instance. Many processed foods, soft drinks, fruits, fruit juices, and drinks contain fructose.

Glucose appears to refuel the muscles better than fructose. Fructose must be processed in the liver before it can contribute to glycogen resynthesis. Glucose, on the other hand, can be used directly for glycogen production without special processing. When comparing fructose and glucose as carbohydrates for refueling, research shows athletes who consume glucose after exercise enjoy a 50 percent faster rate of glycogen resynthesis (over six hours) than those who consume fructose. These results suggest that refueling entirely on high-fructose soft drinks or fruit drinks will hamper your recovery from a tough workout.

5. Drink plenty of fluids for a quick recovery. You lose large amounts of water during exercise, sometimes sweating as much as two quarts per hour. Replacing this lost water during exercise is crucial for performance. After exercise, large amounts of body water must still be replaced, and that requires what I call "active drinking," or drinking fluids beyond feelings of thirst. As a guide, drink a pint of water for every pound of body weight you lose while exercising (weigh yourself before and after a long workout to see the weight difference—you'll be surprised!).

6. Get some rest. Along with carbohydrates and fluids, rest is essential for a speedy recovery and the rebuilding of muscle glycogen. Take time to put your feet up and relax. Stretching, sports massage, or even a soothing bath can help rebuild your muscles for the next strenuous workout.

Follow these six steps for a rapid recovery from exercise and to ready yourself for your next workout or race. Successful performances come not only from hard training but from smart recovery.

AFTER WORK

When your workday comes to an end, more than likely you anticipate your next day's duties and challenge your ability to perform by setting up work goals that require still more effort. But how are you preparing yourself physically for tomorrow's challenges?

Your recovery from a day at work is similar to your recovery from exercise—you need the right pampering, foods, and fluids to recover and rebound quickly for the next day's tasks. As with recovery from exercise, rebuilding from a stress-filled day at work requires choosing foods and fluids wisely. You need not be concerned with eating plates full of carbohydrates, but rather with balancing your recovery meal and resisting performance-sapping foods such as alcohol and caffeine.

Follow my personal plan for a rapid recovery after an exhausting day at work. Your full recharge will mean a productive and energetic tomorrow.

1. Eat a high-carbohydrate, light meal after work. You're tired and looking for a reward for or escape from your efforts at work, but resist eating a dinner that gives nothing back to your body. Aim for a carbohydrate-rich meal with a low-fat protein food, such as pasta, vegetables, and grilled fish. This type of meal replenishes spent energy and vital vitamins and minerals. Even if you leave work late, past dinnertime, still plan on a meal. Keep it light (about 500 to 600 calories) to avoid sluggishness and lack of appetite in the morning. Also, overeating in the evening can contribute to weight gain in some people. See part 2 for after-work meal plans.

2. Make an effort to drink fluids. Chances are you go without taking a break all afternoon and neglect being rehydrated. Make up for needed water by drinking beyond your feeling of thirst. That's right—when you are busy and pressured, your body doesn't tell you adequately about your fluid replacement needs.

3. Resist alcohol for after-work recovery. A ritual for many office workers, after-work drinks can delay your recovery for the next workday. Alcohol saps your performance by affecting brain function and hampering the metabolism of vitamins and minerals crucial to brain and muscle power. Alcohol also drains precious body fluids by acting as a diuretic, increasing water loss through the urine.

In addition to alcohol's effects on the body, after-office drinks preempt the nutritious foods you should be eating. How often have you known someone to let the plan of a well-balanced meal go out the window after a few cocktails. A few drinks on occasion, for relaxation, may not be harmful, but regular use of alcohol limits your ability to recover.

4. Put a limit on "empty" foods. After work, you may be tempted to treat yourself to goodies like premium ice cream, cheesecake, or your favorite cookies. You may even decide to make dessert foods your dinner. But these foods are "empty" when it comes to recovery nutrients. Satisfy your sweet tooth with smaller amounts of goodies and make an effort to postpone desserts until *after* your meal.

5. Keep tabs on caffeine. Resist a coffee pick-me-up after work. Caffeine intake late in the day can mean a poor night's sleep, since caffeine can take six hours or more to clear from the body. A restless night of sleep can leave you stumbling and groggy the next day, particularly by late afternoon when you can't afford a dip in your productivity. Besides coffee and tea, some herbal teas and soft drinks also contain caffeine. Chocolate has a much lower caffeine content, but its effect may still be felt by caffeine-sensitive people. Know when you need to cut off caffeine for the day—8:00 P.M., 4:00 P.M., or maybe nothing after noon—so that you get the rest you need at night.

6. Finish your day with relaxation. Whether you relax and unwind from the day's frenzy with some mindless TV viewing, light reading, or just lying on the floor staring at the ceiling (common for me), it is an important opportunity to begin resting your mind and body, preparing it for the night's sleep. Taking work home and struggling with it until bedtime makes it impossible for most people to truly relax and fall asleep. We noted earlier that your performance, both physical and mental, depends upon your ability to recover and rebuild. Quality rest is an integral part of your recovery.

SWEETNESS: REAL, ARTIFICIAL, OR NONE AT ALL?

It's 3:30 in the afternoon and the hungries have hit again. Digging for change in your pocket, you head for the vending machine to gobble down a sugar pick-me-up. An hour later you've slammed into reverse, you feel light-headed and unable to concentrate, and your workday comes to a fizzling halt.

Can you really blame the sugary candy bar for your performance woes? Yes. For many individuals, eating sugar on an empty stomach can cause swings in blood sugar levels that wreak havoc on performance and stamina. Sugar is also blamed for mood changes, fatigue, hyperactivity in children, obesity, and other evils that have led many people to shun sweets and feel guilty any time sugar passes their lips. How can something so sweet sour your performance?

In all fairness, sugar can be held accountable for only a few health problems. And surprisingly, sweets can routinely be a part of a high-performance diet without sags in stamina. With a little sweet-eats know-how, you can safely satisfy your natural craving for sugar and not be robbed of power nutrients. Understanding how the body handles sugar, when to eat and not eat sweets, where sugar is hidden in foods, and how to use artificial sweeteners will keep you on the performance track.

SUGAR AND ITS ALIASES

Getting a handle on your sugar intake requires some briefing on sugar's many aliases. Sugar is the general term used to describe simple carbohydrates that are made from one or two of the basic sugar units: glucose, fructose, or galactose. No matter whether the sweet you eat is named honey, table sugar, brown sugar, molasses, raw sugar, or corn syrup ... it's sugar. Pick up a packaged food and you'll find several different sugar aliases on the label. Whether you have a bottle of salad dressing or can of soup in hand, chances are it contains sugar, although it may be called something else (see "Sugar in Disguise" on page 76).

WHY DO WE LIKE SWEETS?

There's no doubt about it—we have a national sweet tooth. Our yearly sugar consumption tips in at over 125 pounds per person, and that parcels out to ½ cup of sugar per person each day! Part of our penchant for sweets is inborn. As infants we delight in sweet-tasting fluids. Mother's milk, for instance, is 40 percent sugar (lactose). And as we grow up, our sweet tooth grows with us. Some people have a greater preference for sweets than others. This difference is attributed to environmental influences—how often sweets were eaten and how sweets were used during childhood, many times as a reward and for comforting.

Sugar possesses powerful attributes that, in the opinion of some people, lead to an addiction for sweets. When you eat sugar, you get an immediate reward of a sweet taste, and for some individuals this is extremely pleasurable. Such an immediate positive reinforcement may enhance your craving for sugar. Also, when sugar is paired with another food, broccoli, for instance, your preference for that other food increases.

While it's apparent that we like sugar's taste, a dichotomy exists in the way we think of eating sugary foods. Most of us have grown up being rewarded by a sweet treat for eating nutritionally "correct" food, like vegetables. Yet many authorities condemn eating sugar, and we feel guilty when we indulge. Throughout our lives the reward for doing "right" is to eat something "wrong." No wonder we have a love/hate relationship with sugar.

HOW YOUR BODY HANDLES SUGAR

No matter what type of sugar you eat, your body quickly processes it into glucose—the basic unit used by virtually all cells in your body. The speed at which sugar is absorbed has both advantages and drawbacks. A shot of sugar from fruit juice or hard candy can surge into the bloodstream within minutes, which is good for quick energy needs, such as during exercise. But this speedy absorption is not so good during those times when a steady supply of carbohydrate energy is needed—a long afternoon at work, for example.

Remember, from our earlier discussion of carbohydrates, how the body works hard to maintain a constant blood sugar level? After a sugar snack, the high blood sugar level is brought back

SUGAR IN DISGUISE

These terms commonly appear on food labels, but each is just another name for sugar. Don't be fooled by a label that reads "sugar-free"—the product may not contain sucrose (common table sugar) but can have other added sugars.

Brown sugar: Refined white sugar sprayed with, or crystalized with, molasses.

Confectioner's sugar: Finely ground white sugar (sucrose).

Corn syrup: A liquid made from enzymatic digestion of cornstarch into refined sugars—glucose and maltose, with small pieces of starch. Used in soft drinks and packaged foods.

Dextrin: Small pieces of starch made of a few glucose units.

Dextrose: Another name for glucose. When added to foods it is usually made from the complete digestion of cornstarch.

Fructose: Found in fruits and honey; sweeter tasting than table sugar.

Glucose: The principal carbohydrate found in blood and nearly all plant foods.

Honey: Composed of fructose, glucose, water, and a small amount of sucrose; tastes sweeter than table sugar and has 22 calories per teaspoon (versus 16 calories per teaspoon of table sugar).

Maltose: Commonly called malt sugar; made from fermentation and digestion of starch; found in beer, breads, and sprouted seeds.

Mannitol: A sugar alcohol half as sweet as sugar; used as a caloric substitute for sucrose; large amounts cause diarrhea.

Maple syrup: The sap from rock maple trees, composed of sucrose, water, and small amounts of fructose and glucose.

Molasses: Syrup left over after sucrose has been crystal-

(continued)

Sugar—*Continued*

lized from sugar cane or sugar beets.

Natural sweeteners: A term used to describe sugar made from "natural" sources—any of the sweeteners listed here are natural.

Raw sugar: Truly "raw" sugar is unfit to eat due to soil and bacterial contamination.

Sorbitol: A sugar alcohol half as sweet as sugar and more slowly absorbed into the body; used as a sweetener in foods for diabetics.

Sucrose: Common table sugar made from sugar cane or sugar beets, composed of glucose and fructose.

Turbinado sugar: Similar to brown sugar; made from crystallized sucrose that is partly refined (sometimes called raw sugar, though technically it is not).

Xylitol: A sugar alcohol equal in sweetness to sucrose; when used in place of sucrose it reduces the incidence of cavities.

to a normal level through the action of insulin, a hormone that allows glucose to enter body cells.

In some people insulin does its job too well, and blood sugar levels fall below normal. This is called hypoglycemia, and it can bring on dizziness, shaking, hunger, and rapid heartbeat. Many individuals self-diagnose hypoglycemia when they feel light-headed after eating a candy bar. Consuming a large amount of sugar after a few days on a low-carbohydrate diet can cause these hypoglycemic symptoms. However, true hypoglycemia occurs in very few people.

The only way to diagnose hypoglycemia is through a special blood test, administered following a measured sugar load. If you feel low blood sugar may be what's troubling your performance, see your physician, since this problem could represent a serious medical condition.

After the glucose from a sugary snack enters your body's tissues, it can be used immediately for energy or stored as glyco-gen in the muscles and liver for later use, during exercise or when you've gone without food for many hours.

However, since so much sugar is available at once, your body tends to convert some of this extra glucose into fat. Remember, your body stores a limited supply of energy as sugar. Fat transformation happens in the liver, and the fat is then transported into the blood and eventually to your fat stores—around your waist, for instance. Those people who already have a high blood fat level must control sugar in their diet to avoid further problems.

Also, the sugar fructose converts more readily into fat than glucose does, so it can dangerously elevate blood fat levels. This fat-boosting action of fructose is of real concern because of the increasing use of high-fructose corn sweetener in soft drinks and other processed foods. Sweetened beverages alone account for 32 percent of our sugar intake, with much of this sugar as fructose.

Sugar primarily serves as an energy source for your body—and that's it, nothing more. In fact, sugar is virtually 100 percent pure carbohydrate, which means it provides zero in the way of vitamins and minerals needed to process this sugar energy. Some people mistakenly choose honey, thinking it contains B vitamins and minerals needed to process this sugar. However, honey contains an insignificant amount of these nutrients—less than 8 percent of what's needed for metabolizing this sugar. Simply put, sugar robs you of vital performance nutrients and it does so in two ways.

1. When you eat sugar, it displaces more nutritious foods in the diet.

2. Sugar requires vitamins and minerals for its metabolism, which most sugary foods don't provide.

HOW BAD IS SUGAR FOR YOUR HEALTH AND YOUR PERFORMANCE?

While sugar certainly can be blamed for robbing you of precious nutrients, there are few other evils truly attributable to sweets alone. Some health- and performance-related problems, such as feelings of fatigue or changes in mood, may be linked to sugar for some people. Yet I invite you to take a look at the big health picture. The facts may calm your worries and subdue your guilt about eating sugar in moderation. Now learn the real story on sugar and:

□ Fatigue. You may feel sleepy and tired (not weak) after a

sugary snack. It has a calming effect in some people because it facilitates the release of the soothing brain chemical serotonin. This happens particularly in early afternoon, when a normal performance dip occurs.

- Hypoglycemia. This is unlikely for a vast majority of people. True hypoglycemia, low blood sugar, has other causes. Yet a large sugar dose after days of eating a low-carbohydrate diet may produce similar symptoms.

- Mood changes/hyperactivity. Scientific studies have repeatedly absolved sugar as the cause of hyperactivity in children or of any aggressive behavior in adults. While many parents and teachers feel there is a link between sugar and behavior problems, sugar has been shown to have the opposite effect, a calming influence.

- Diabetes. While sugar must be tightly controlled in a diabetic's diet since there is an inability to handle glucose, sugar itself does not cause this disorder.

- Obesity. Weight gain can't be blamed on sugar alone. Too many calories, particularly from fat, cause excess body fat storage. Many high-sugar foods are also high in fat and thus play a part in weight problems. But obesity is a complex condition, with both food and behavior as contributing factors.

- Cancer. No form of sugar has been linked to cancer. Yet because eating more fruits, vegetables, and grains may reduce your cancer risk, eating too much sugar may preempt these important foods in your diet.

- Cavities. Yes. Tooth decay is perhaps sugar's most blatant health problem. Sticky sweets and sugared drinks are the worst offenders among causes of tooth decay. Regular brushing and flossing, along with eating sweets with meals rather than between meals, helps control cavities.

- Heart disease. The case against sugar as a dietary risk factor for heart disease is weak. However, certain people with already high levels of blood triglyceride (fat) and cholesterol should limit sugar intake, particularly fructose found in honey, soft drinks, processed foods, and fruits.

EAT SWEETS THE RIGHT WAY

If you're like most Americans, your sweet tooth needs taming. You should get no more than 10 percent of your calories from sugar, which is half of the present average intake. Cutting your sugar intake in half will make room for other foods packed with power nutrients. But to say you'll do without any sugar is not only impractical, it goes against your natural craving for sweets. You can have your cake and eat it, too, by following my guidelines for eating sweets safely.

Limit your sugar intake. Stay ahead in the stamina game by eating a diet packed with complex carbohydrates, instead of a high-sugar diet low in vitamins, minerals, and fiber. Control your intake by limiting sugared soft drinks plus sugar in coffee and tea and on cereal, all of which account for 50 percent of our total sugar intake. Be familiar with sugar's many disguises (see "Sugar in Disguise" on page 76) when buying packaged foods, and read labels.

Avoid high-sugar foods as snacks. Consuming a sugary candy bar or drink may leave you feeling less than energetic an hour later. Some people suffer a "sugar low"—dizziness, shaking, light-headedness—after eating sweets, while others notice no ill effects. Keep track of your experiences with sugary snacks and know when to say no to a sugar treat. Have canned vegetable juice, whole-grain crackers, or bread on hand for an energy pick-me-up.

Eat your sweets after meals. When eaten along with complex carbs, protein, and fat (as in a meal of chicken, potato, and salad with dressing), sugar is released into the bloodstream more slowly. Eating sweets after a meal also helps control how much sugar you eat. You may be able to devour a dozen cookies or more as a snack, but you probably won't want to eat that many right after a meal.

Switch to low-sugar sweets. You can lessen your preference for highly sweetened foods by gradually switching over to sweets that are less intense. Top your ice cream with fruit instead of sweet syrup or candy toppings; choose breakfast cereals lower in sugar (check the label); combine a sweet with fruit for an overall lower sugar intake (two cookies and an orange instead of four cookies alone); dilute fruit or sugared drinks with soda water.

Watch for foods with hidden sugar. Surprisingly, many foods that you would least suspect of it have added sugar. Along with other sweets, these foods can boost your total sugar intake beyond desired levels. Here's a list of some foods with hidden sugar:

☐ Breakfast cereals
☐ Canned beans
☐ Canned fruit
☐ Canned soups
☐ Catsup
☐ Flavored milk
☐ Luncheon meats
☐ Muffin and pancake mixes
☐ Spaghetti sauce (commercial)
☐ Specialty breads (e.g., raisin bread)
☐ TV dinners

Cut back on the sugar in recipes. Most cookie, cake, and pie recipes fare well when sugar is cut back by one-third. For treats even lower in sugar, use specially modified recipes, since decreasing the sugar content too much without guidance will change the texture and color of baked goods. You may also want to try recipes that call for molasses, which contains a fair amount of iron and calcium, although its strong flavor limits its uses in many recipes.

Switch over to fresh and dried fruit for dessert. A juicy piece of fruit can really satisfy a sweet tooth, and you get vitamins, minerals, fiber, and virtually no fat to boot. Dried fruit, also loaded with nutrients and fat-free, can be intensely sweet (high in fructose). Remember to brush your teeth after eating dried fruit, since it can stick to your teeth and encourage cavity development.

SWEETENING ARTIFICIALLY

Everything from soft drinks to frozen desserts is available with artificial sweeteners, allowing you to bypass sugar's calories and tooth decay risk. You can take advantage of artificial sweeteners if you understand the best way to use them in your diet. For example, if you satisfy your sweet cravings with sugar substitutes, you make room for performance foods such as complex carbohydrates.

WHAT ARE ARTIFICIAL SWEETENERS?

Sugar substitutes comprise a rapidly growing billion-dollar industry. These substances, generally calorie free and many times sweeter than sugar, have various uses in foods and beverages. The major artificial sweeteners are:

Aspartame (NutraSweet). Made from two amino acids (protein) and approximately 200 times sweeter than sugar, it is the most widely used sugar substitute. Because of its chemical structure, however, aspartame loses its sweetening power when it's heated, limiting its use in desserts and baked goods. Aspartame is used primarily in beverages, frozen desserts, other non-baked sweet goods, and as a tabletop sweetener (sprinkled into coffee, tea, or on cereal).

Sucralose (Splenda). This is common table sugar chemically altered to make it 600 times sweeter. Unlike aspartame, sucralose doesn't break down during baking. This means it can substitute for sugar in cookies, cakes, and pies as well as in beverages, frozen desserts, and as a tabletop sweetener.

Acesulfame K (Sunette). This is similar to aspartame in sweetening power but more stable, so it can be used in baked goods. As with saccharin, some criticize its aftertaste.

Saccharin (Sweet 'n Low; Sucaryl). Made from petroleum-based products and 300 times sweeter than sugar, saccharin's generally used as a tabletop sweetener. Aspartame (now accounting for 70 percent of all artificial sweetener use) has replaced saccharin in beverages.

While safety concerns will always surround artificial sweeteners, all these sugar substitutes are approved for use in the United States by the Food and Drug Administration. Aspartame, for instance, was the most heavily tested artificial sweetener in history. Cyclamate, a sugar substitute banned in 1969 as a cancer threat, will reappear on the market due to new testing that shows it is safe for consumption.

WHAT ARTIFICIAL SWEETENERS CAN AND CAN'T DO FOR YOU

Substituting for sugar, these sweeteners save you calories. They convert a can of sugary soft drink from 160 calories to 1 calorie. Frozen desserts and baked goods made with sugar substitutes have calorie savings of about 30 percent. Passing up sugar's calories makes room for other foods, like complex carbohydrates, that you might otherwise have done without.

Used reasonably, artificial sweeteners save calories and allow you to make sensible choices at meals. An artificially sweetened beverage along with a meal or snack, for example, saves about 150 calories. In theory, this would allow you to eat an extra bagel, a large baked potato, or two pieces of fruit—all loaded

TABLE 2-12 *HIGH-SUGAR TRADE-OFFS*

Instead of . . .	Choose . . .
Sugar-sweetened fruit yogurt	Sugar-free fruit flavored yogurt with: 1 whole-grain roll *or* 2 rice cakes *or* ½ cup hot cereal *or* 1 peach *or* 1½ cups sliced strawberries
Sugar-sweetened pudding, or ice cream	Sugar-free pudding, or ice cream and: extra serving of steamed vegetables and small dinner roll *or* ½ cup cooked pasta *or* tossed green salad with low-cal dressing *or* large piece of fruit
Sugared soda or other sugar-sweetened drink	Diet soda, or artificially sweetened lemonade fruit drink or iced tea, along with: 3 cups air-popped popcorn *or* 4 rice cakes *or* 1 bagel *or* 6 whole-grain crackers and 1 orange *or* 1 banana and 1 slice wheat bread *or* 1½ cup whole-grain cereal *or* 1 slice corn bread and 1 apple

with vitamins, minerals, and smooth-burning complex carbohy-drates.

Needless to say, this is not the way most of us use artificial sweeteners. In fact, since sugar substitutes have been in use, there has been no thinning of our national profile as a whole. Many researchers criticize the way artificial sweeteners are pro-moted—fooling the public into believing that products con-taining them cause weight loss.

In fact, a handful of research reports suggest that artificial sweeteners may not contribute to weight loss at all, but actually cause weight gain! The theory is that users may want to eat more to compensate (psychologically and physiologically) for the cal-ories they "missed" by using sugar substitutes.

However, these few studies focused on saccharin. Studies performed with aspartame showed different results. In experi-mental studies carried out at the University of Toronto, aspar-tame ingested one hour before a buffet lunch did not influence the amount of food the subjects ate. Additionally, a Harvard University study showed that obese women who consumed aspartame-containing foods during a 12-week weight-reduction program lost an average 16.5 pounds. That was about 4 pounds more than the average weight loss for women in the study whose diet didn't include sugar substitutes but contained the same number of calories.

The value of artificial sweeteners as a diet aid is controversial at best. However, you can benefit from the calorie savings in sugar substitutes. Using artificial sweeteners the *right* way is the key.

CHAPTER **3**

PERFORMANCE PROTEIN

When you hear the word *protein,* what comes to mind? A well-muscled body builder drinking a protein shake, or perhaps a hulking football player devouring a huge steak? You probably don't think yourself capable of benefiting from more red meat or other protein-rich foods; if anything you should cut back . . . right?

Wrong! Your body depends upon incoming protein from food for daily performance. And you may not be getting enough. A lingering cold, chronic fatigue, or general weakness are just a few of the signs that indicate you may be short on protein. Beyond making muscle, protein foods give you the right stuff to fight off disease; to build, repair, and maintain all types of tissue in your body; to keep brain cells thinking and blood flowing. You require a steady supply of protein to meet day-to-day peak performance demands. Even more high-quality protein is necessary with exercise, since body protein breaks down during a workout or any other heavy muscular activity.

You must know what your body needs for lasting power at work or during a workout. With my Protein Primer, I show you the top protein foods for good health and hustle. I also give you the facts on red meat and the lowdown on protein and amino acid pills, powders, and potions. I simplify vegetarian eating and show you how to plan a semi-meatless menu for added health benefits.

YOU MAY NEED MORE PROTEIN

One case history will help clarify a typical protein problem. Jim, a cameraman with an erratic schedule, had a protein dilemma. Much to his amazement, Jim wasn't eating enough protein. As an avid runner, he realized the importance of carbohydrates, so most of his meals were actually snacks consisting of cereals, breads, fruits, and crackers, with only an occasional dinner of chicken or fish (once or twice a week).

I spoke with Jim after he had a disappointing few months of training, coupled with extreme fatigue at work and colds that seemed to last for weeks. I complimented him on his carbohydrate intake but told him his protein level was dangerously low. At less than 35 grams a day, it was about half of his requirement. This suboptimal protein intake helped explain Jim's chronic illness and fatigue.

A few simple changes—skim milk on his cereal, water-packed tuna with salads at lunch, and bean-rice dishes for dinner—bumped up Jim's protein intake to a healthful 80 grams daily. Within a few weeks, Jim's performance at work was more vigorous, with energy left to squeeze in his daily runs, schedule permitting.

You may be facing the same protein deficit Jim did. Sporadic eating and less-than-routine work schedules often put the square meal concept on the back burner, risking a low protein intake. I find that the people who typically don't eat enough protein are those with crazy schedules who end up grazing their way through the day on carbs—breads, fruit, and cereal—while skipping out on protein-rich foods. Use my Protein Primer to find out if you're eating enough protein (or too much) and to learn why protein is so vital for your performance.

PROTEIN PRIMER

As we learned in chapter 1, most of our body is water. Take away that water, however, and what's left is mostly protein, thousands of different proteins, giving your body brain power, muscle power, and disease-fighting power.

Every cell in your body has protein. In fact, many different proteins with their specific duties enable your entire body to function smoothly. Your body makes these specific proteins by breaking down the bulk protein in the food you eat into its components, called amino acids. Your body arranges these amino acids in thousands of different combinations to create each kind of protein needed to power nearly everything you do.

Amino acids are like the letters of the alphabet. By themselves, they have little meaning, but when linked together properly they form specific words (proteins) which do have meaning. And like the 26 letters in the alphabet, the 20 different amino acids can be arranged and rearranged for various purposes. Think of the words *proteins* and *pointers* made from the same eight letters, with completely different meanings because the sequence of those letters is different.

Amino acid sequencing is responsible for the thousands of different proteins that keep your body running—on the job or while working out. Proteins give your body:
□ Structure, shape, and definition
□ Resistance to disease
□ Ability to repair and maintain tissue
□ Hormones to control metabolism
□ Energy

Each day your body loses protein in the form of hair, skin, and nails, along with protein that is routinely broken down in the body. To keep up with these demands, your body needs a daily supply of amino acids from foods. However, you can actually get by with ingesting only 9 of the 20 different amino acids. These 9 are called essential, meaning that since your body can't manufacture them, it is essential you get them from your diet. The remaining amino acids are made quite easily by the body, given a necessary building block—the element nitrogen.

FOOD PROTEIN

These essential amino acids are irreplaceable—which explains your need for daily protein intake, ideally at all meals. Food protein supplies you with essential amino acids and the nitrogen you need to make your own protein. Be it steak or tofu, foods containing protein usually have all or almost all 20 amino acids.

But how much of each essential amino acid that a food has is crucial? Food proteins that have all nine amino acids in the right proportions, meeting body needs, are called complete proteins. Incomplete proteins, on the other hand, are deficient in one or more of the nine essentials, falling short on some parts you need to build body proteins. Just as you can't spell a word without the necessary letters, you can't make specific proteins in your body if you don't have the essential amino acids.

Meat, milk, eggs, fish, and poultry (animal products) are examples of complete proteins. In fact, the most complete or "perfect" protein is in egg whites. You also eat many incomplete protein grains—wheat, corn, oats, rye, rice, barley; dried beans (legumes)—kidney, garbanzo, pinto, soybeans; and nuts and seeds—sunflower, sesame, peanuts, and almonds. But these incomplete proteins can easily be combined with others to make complete proteins.

Combining incomplete proteins balances out the nine essential amino acids you need for top health. It just so happens that certain incomplete protein foods complement others. Grains, like corn, are low in an essential amino acid called lysine, yet dried beans have plenty of lysine. But beans are low in another essential amino acid, methionine, while grains are not. Put these two incomplete proteins together (as in a bean burrito) and you have a complete protein combination that is not deficient in any of the nine essential amino acids. This process of combining incomplete proteins allows vegetarians (people who do not eat meats, milk products, or eggs) to fill their protein requirements. More on vegetarian and semivegetarian eating styles is coming up later in this chapter.

The general rule for combining proteins is that virtually all grains complement and complete the proteins in beans (legumes). Also, whenever you combine grains or beans with a complete protein (milk, meats, eggs), you complement the incomplete protein (grains or beans), increasing the overall protein value of the combination. Pouring milk over cereal or mixing tuna with rice, for instance, makes up for any amino acid deficiencies in the cereal or rice.

Table 3-1 *POWERFUL PROTEIN COMBINATIONS*

Basic Pairs	Specific Foods
Legumes and grains	Baked beans and brown bread
	Lentil soup and rye bread
	Pinto beans and corn tortillas
	Refried beans and rice
	Tofu and Chinese noodles
Legumes and seeds	Garbanzo beans and sunflower seeds
	Soybeans and sesame seeds

HOW YOUR BODY HANDLES PROTEIN

After you eat a juicy steak or tofuburger, the food proteins are broken down into individual amino acids by your body so it can recombine these subparts into its own proteins. The breakdown process begins when a mouthful of food lands in your stomach, where gastric juices, containing acid and enzymes, split food proteins into shorter chains of amino acids.

This partially digested protein then passes into your small intestine, where other enzymes, called peptidases, split the amino acid chain into individual amino acids. Protein digestion is like separating the letters in a word: The word no longer exists—just a mixture of letters. Individual amino acid molecules, of which there are millions from all sorts of food proteins and recycled body proteins, then pass through your intestinal wall and into your bloodstream.

I want to interject at this point that amino acids, whether from food, recycled body protein, or a packaged amino acid or protein supplement, are indistinguishable from each other. Once in your intestinal tract, amino acids are biochemically and nutritionally identical, regardless of the source of protein or the form in which it was eaten.

Once in the bloodstream, there are four paths an amino acid can take. It can be:

□ Used directly to make a body protein: muscle, skin, hormones, or antibodies, for instance.
□ Converted into another amino acid that the body may need.
□ Used to make other chemicals in the body, like brain chemicals.
□ Used for energy.

Thus, not all the amino acids from foods go directly into making muscles or hormones. What your body does with each individual amino acid depends upon what's happening in your body at the time you eat. Your body can't store protein for later use as it stores carbohydrate or fat. For this reason, protein must be used efficiently as it comes into the bloodstream and tissues. When amino acids enter your bloodstream, their use (any of the four possibilities above) is determined by a priority system your body has established to ensure survival and maximum performance.

Tops on the priority list is the critical demand of your brain and muscles for carbohydrate energy. If you have short-changed yourself on calories, your body will divert incoming amino acids for energy needs.

Additionally, some amino acids may need to be transformed into carbohydrate to power your brain and muscles if you're skimping on dietary carbs or running low on glycogen during exercise. Spending amino acids this way is costly and inefficient for your body—it's only an emergency backup system. This process pulls amino acids away from their job of making up proteins in your body—thereby sapping your performance and potentially weakening your defenses against illness. For example, very-low-calorie diets or starvation, common ways people go about losing weight, can cause muscle and organ tissues to lose valuable body proteins that must be replaced. Frequently, people who go long periods without sufficient food energy from carbohydrates or protein find themselves plagued with illness and fatigue.

HOW MUCH PROTEIN DO YOU NEED?

All of this brings up some serious questions: How much protein is enough? Is more protein always better? If you exercise or train regularly, or face demanding stress at work, how does protein fit into the performance factor?

For starters, an official Recommended Dietary Allowance (RDA) for protein exists: 0.8 grams of protein per kilogram of body weight. This is the same as 0.36 grams of protein per pound of body weight. Using the RDA, this works out to be 47 grams for a 130-pound woman (equivalent to three ounces of broiled fish, 1½ cups of lentils and rice, and 1 cup of yogurt) and 66 grams for a 170-pound man (found in six ounces of roasted chicken, 1½ cups of skim milk, and one baked potato).

You can figure your own protein requirement by multiplying your body weight in pounds by 0.36 (roughly speaking, your numerical protein requirement in grams is approximately one-third of your body weight in pounds).

As background, the RDA does not represent a minimum standard but instead a level of protein that has a built-in safety factor, calculated to meet the needs of virtually all healthy people in the population. So when you calculate your requirement, realize this is designed to actually exceed what you need.

EXERCISE DEMANDS ARE SPECIAL

It sounds simple so far, but some researchers think the RDA for protein is still not enough for certain individuals. Hard-training athletes, for example, may need more. Various studies with different athletic types—runners and weight lifters alike—suggest that the RDA does fall short of meeting their protein need for optimal performance. Additionally, boosting protein intake while on low-calorie diets may help prevent protein breakdown and help replace body proteins that are being used for energy.

In one study, for example, men who did aerobic exercise regularly (biking, running, swimming) needed additional protein—50 percent over their RDA. By measuring nitrogen balance, a technique used to determine if more protein is lost from the body than is taken in through the diet, the researchers found these active men needed additional protein to cover losses due to exercise. The difference amounted to about 27 grams (for a 150-pound person). In terms of food, that translates to 2½ cups of milk, three ounces of chicken, or 2½ cups of beans and rice.

The explanation for this increased protein need comes from numerous studies showing amino acids are broken down for energy in exercising muscles. So in effect, proteins are burned along with carbs and fats to supply you with energy. How much energy the protein supplies depends on how long you exercise and how much glycogen is stored in your muscles.

During an hour-long exercise session, only 5 percent of the energy comes from protein breakdown. However, protein must supply 10 to 15 percent of the energy required when glycogen stores are drained during exercise sessions of two or more hours. This means that, during exercise, you break down a bit of muscle, which needs rebuilding during post-exercise recovery.

For strength athletes, such as weight lifters, protein needs may also be pushed up, but only slightly—10 to 20 percent. This extra protein goes to increases in muscle weight rather than energy use. An extra ten grams of protein daily over the RDA, or less than two ounces of chicken, covers the increase. However, it must be pointed out that not all research with this type of athlete supports the theory that extra protein quickly makes bigger muscles. Some research finds that strength athletes are even more efficient with protein and that they may be able to get away with actually eating less, leaving more room for energizing carbs.

WORKDAY PROTEIN NEEDS

What is true for the athlete is almost certainly true for the stressed businessperson. As you strive to maximize performance at work, particularly during long working days or while on the road, protein needs are most likely met with the RDA. However, if you cut back on calories to drop weight or because of a time crunch, additional protein is needed. Try to eat enough protein daily to meet your RDA, plus an additional 10 percent to maximize your work performance.

To be really covered, *I recommend eating protein at a level of the RDA plus an additional 25 percent*. This will more than match your needs—both at work and for working out. But for those of you involved in heavy training (two-plus hours daily), tack 50 percent onto the RDA to cover protein losses. Check Table 3-2 to determine your best protein level.

MEASURE YOUR PERSONAL PROTEIN REQUIREMENTS

The debate about how much protein an active person needs is largely academic—most of us consume one-and-a-half to two times our RDA. At this level of protein intake, any increased needs due to exercise or daily work stress are more than covered.

Some people, however, may be eating a low-protein diet. If you're a meat-and-potatoes diner, fast-food fan, or a serious vegetarian, chances are you're doing just fine, at least with regard to protein needs. It's the quasi-vegetarians or carbohydrate-over-doer types that may be falling short on protein and risking a performance-sapping diet. While carbs are crucial for lasting energy at work and during a workout, going overboard can mean you're bumping out protein.

You can use Table 3-3 to check up on your protein intake. Once you know how much protein you need from Table 3-2, compare a day's worth of eating with the values in Table 3-3 and see how you're doing.

TOO MUCH OF A GOOD THING

You require protein in your diet on a daily basis to replace the protein and amino acids that are constantly being broken down and lost. But if you eat more protein, will this give you a jump on upcoming needs or make bigger and better muscles? Hardly. Extra protein in the diet, beyond what your body demands for rebuilding and repair, does not go to make extra muscle, to make you more resistant to illnesses, or to help you grow stronger fingernails. You can't store protein for later use, as you can carbohydrate and fat. Your body must use, transform, or discard the protein on the spot. If your body gets more protein (amino acids) than it needs, the extra is broken down and stored as fat or used for energy.

Table 3-2 *PROTEIN NEEDS*

Use this chart to determine how much protein you need daily. The protein RDA should meet the needs of most people. Tack on 10 percent with activity and an extra 25 or 50 percent if you exercise heavily each day.

Body Weight (lb.)	RDA	RDA + 10%	RDA + 25%	RDA + 50%
110	40	44	50	60
120	43	47	54	62
130	47	52	59	70
140	50	55	63	75
150	54	59	68	81
160	58	64	72	87
170	61	67	76	92
180	65	71	81	97
190	68	75	85	102
200	72	79	90	108
210	76	84	95	114
220	79	87	99	119

SOURCE: National Academy of Sciences, *Recommended Dietary Allowances* (Washington, D.C.: National Academy Press, 1989).

This process of handling surplus protein from the diet has negative side effects. The liver and kidneys must process the unwanted nitrogen from surplus amino acids. Your kidneys have to flush it out in the urine, so you need greater water intake and you risk the debilitating effects of dehydration. Additionally, overdoing protein may cause loss of calcium in the urine—a particular concern for women and others at risk for osteoporosis, who do not get enough calcium in their diet.

While routinely eating a high-protein diet makes the kidneys work overtime, there is a lack of evidence that otherwise healthy people eating too much protein have kidney problems. If you eat 50 percent to even 100 percent over the RDA for protein,

Table 3-3 *PROTEIN COUNTER*

You probably need between 45 and 90 grams of protein daily (depending upon your body weight). Here's where you get it. Add up your protein count. Are you over or under?

Food	Portion	Protein (g)	Calories
Beans and Grains			
Bread	2 slices	3	160
Cereal, ready-to-eat	1 cup	2	110
Garbanzo beans	1 cup	15	270
Lentils	1 cup	18	231
Pasta	1 cup	5	160
Pinto beans	1 cup	14	235
Potato, baked, with skin	1	5	212
Rice, brown	1 cup	5	232
Soybeans	1 cup	28	298
Tempeh (soybean product)	½ cup	16	165
Tofu	½ cup	10	94
Dairy Products			
Cheddar or Swiss cheese	1 oz.	7	110
Cottage cheese, low-fat	½ cup	14	82
Ice cream	1 cup	5	270
Milk, skim or low-fat	8 oz.	8	86/120
Mozzarella, low-fat	1 oz.	7	72
Yogurt, plain, low-fat	1 cup	10	160
Meat, Poultry, Fish, and Eggs			
Beef, top round, broiled	3 oz.	26	180
Chicken, light meat, roasted, no skin	3 oz.	26	150
Egg	1 large	6	80
Egg whites	2	7	32
Ground beef, lean, cooked	3 oz.	21	214
Pork loin, roasted	3 oz.	28	234
Salmon, broiled	3 oz.	23	157

(continued)

Table 3-3—*Continued*

Food	Portion	Protein (g)	Calories
Meat, Poultry, Fish, and Eggs			
Snapper, broiled	3 oz.	23	109
Tuna, water-packed	3 oz.	25	111
Turkey, dark-meat, roasted, no skin	3 oz.	25	160
Veal roast, broiled	3 oz.	23	184

SOURCE: Adapted from J. A. T. Pennington, *Bowes and Church's Food Values of Portions Commonly Used*, 15th ed. (Philadelphia: J. B. Lippincott, 1989).

you're safe as far as kidney health is concerned. However, if you take protein supplements, you're headed for trouble.

Excessive protein intake (five or more times the RDA), usually due to the heavy use of protein supplements, can cause a loss of bone calcium via the urine. This calcium loss is particularly dangerous for women who are at risk for the debilitating disease osteoporosis. Also, consuming too much protein can lead to dehydration, since so much of the water we drink is utilized in excreting protein wastes in the urine.

Even more unwanted baggage comes along with eating too much protein—fat and cholesterol. Most protein rich-foods we typically select—meats, eggs, cheese—are high in fat, particularly cholesterol-elevating saturated fats. And depending on how we prepare these foods, by frying or with creamy sauces, the fat content can even climb higher. Animal products like these also supply a dose of cholesterol you may want to avoid for the sake of cardiovascular health.

In the next chapter, I discuss the fats that are good or bad for top performance. For now, compare the top ten protein foods in Table 3-4 with your standard protein fare. I recommend these choices to executives and athletes alike. These selections are low in fat and cholesterol and pack additional power nutrients like iron and zinc. Remember that vegetable sources of protein are cholesterol free and typically lower in fat than most animal foods, while supplying generous amounts of the carbs you need for stamina. Your goal is simple: Meet your protein needs without taking in the extra fat that saps your performance.

Making the switch to more healthful protein choices requires a few simple substitutions. Whether you're at a fast-food outlet, a fine restaurant, or at home preparing a six-minute meal, you can make the most of protein foods without getting what you don't want. Follow the list of substitutions in Table 3-5 for better health and performance. Also, check chapter 8 for ways to work your menu while at home or on the road, getting the protein you need to be at your best.

VEGETARIAN EATING: BENEFITS, CAUTIONS, AND HOW-TO'S

Do vegetarians make better runners, better executives, better citizens? People often quiz me on the benefits of vegetarianism and wonder whether they can improve their work performance, athletic performance, or even their overall health by going meatless.

Lower risk for intestinal cancer, heart disease, and osteoporosis, lower blood pressure, and perhaps greater ease at maintaining your weight are some of the benefits that may await you with a pure vegetarian eating style that is low in fat, rich in performance-boosting carbohydrates, and high in fiber. There is one catch, though—you have to know how to follow a vegetarian eating style in a healthful way. Unless you stick to some basic rules, this type of eating has potentially damaging side effects that can leave you with less than the full strength you need to meet your daily challenges.

Choosing beans and rice over meats can, in fact, be an advantageous dietary change for an active person. But good health and better performance are not foolproof results of a meatless diet. The fact is, a meatless diet and one containing meat can be equally healthful—or equally unhealthful. The nutritional success of vegetarianism or any other kind of diet depends on individual planning.

Basic to any diet is the need for:
□ Adequate protein to supply nutritionally essential amino acids.
□ Nitrogen to replenish body proteins.

(continued on page 101)

Table 3-4 *TOP TEN PROTEIN FOODS FOR HEALTH AND HUSTLE*

Here are my best picks for quality protein along with power nutrients you need for top performance.

Food	Calories	Protein (g)	Calories from Fat (%)	Plus . . .
1. 3 oz. broiled fresh tuna	157	25	30	214% USRDA vitamin A 154% USRDA vitamin B$_{12}$ 45% USRDA niacin Good source of omega-3's
2. 1½ cups lentils and rice	347	17	3	77% carbohydrate calories 8 grams of fiber 31% USRDA iron 13% USRDA zinc 19% USRDA copper 67% USRDA folate
3. 1 cup nonfat yogurt	127	13	3	45% USRDA calcium 31% USRDA riboflavin 23% USRDA vitamin B$_{12}$ 15% USRDA zinc
4. 3 oz. steamed clams	126	22	12	1400% USRDA vitamin B$_{12}$ 132% USRDA iron 15% USRDA zinc 29% USRDA copper

Food	Calories	Protein (g)	Nutrients
5. 3 oz. lean beef, top round	164	27	14% USRDA iron (heme iron)* 32% USRDA zinc 24% USRDA vitamin B$_6$ 26% USRDA niacin 35% USRDA vitamin B$_{12}$
6. 3 oz. roasted chicken breast	150	26	53% USRDA niacin 26% USRDA vitamin B$_6$
7. 1 cup pinto beans and two tortillas	369	16	9 grams of fiber 74% USRDA folate 40% USRDA iron 17% USRDA zinc 22% USRDA copper
8. 3 oz. broiled salmon	157	23	95% USRDA vitamin B$_{12}$ Excellent source of omega-3's 29% USRDA niacin
9. 3 oz. roasted dark-meat turkey	160	25	26% USRDA zinc 11% USRDA iron (heme iron)*
10. ½ cup firm tofu and baked potato	300	24	56% USRDA copper 87% USRDA iron

SOURCE: Adapted from J. A. T. Pennington, *Bowes and Church's Food Values of Portions Commonly Used*, 15th ed. (Philadelphia: J. B. Lippincott, 1989).

A well-absorbed form of iron.

Table 3-5 *GOOD-FOR-YOU PROTEIN TIPS*

Try these easy-to-do substitutions and tips for healthful protein foods.

Instead of . . .	Try . . .
Choosing higher-fat beef cuts such as ribs (prime), choice sirloin, flank, or brisket	Picking lean beef cuts such as top round, round tip, sirloin, tenderloin
Using bottled marinades with oil	Marinating meats in herbs and wine or lemon juice
Cooking with skin on poultry and visible fat on meat	Partially freezing poultry and meat to easily remove skin and trim visible fat
Using cream cheese or mayonnaise	Spreading peanut butter or cottage cheese blended with yogurt on bagels and muffins
Using higher-fat cheeses such as cheddar, Monterey jack, and Swiss	Choosing low-fat cheese or "lite" processed cheese
Adding oil, butter, or margarine for cooking meats	Sautéing and browning meat or tofu in a nonstick skillet
Adding fat to stews, soups, sauces	Skimming fat off
Frying or roasting meat or poultry in a pan	Broiling or roasting on an oven rack
Panfrying or breading fish	Poaching, broiling, or microwaving
Using 2 whole eggs	Using 1 egg white and one large egg
Choosing pastrami, bologna and salami	Picking lean ham, thin sliced roast beef and turkey as deli choices

□ Sufficient energy to meet the caloric demands of exercise.
□ Various essential vitamins and minerals.

A diet that excludes all or some animal products (meat, milk, eggs) requires certain modifications to meet these basic needs. But the extent of modification depends upon the type of vegetarian you become. The most common types are:

□ "Vegans," or strict vegetarians—eat no animal products.
□ Lacto-ovo vegetarians—use dairy products (lacto-) and eggs (ovo-).
□ "New" or "semi" vegetarians—eat fish (pescovegetarian) or poultry (poulovegetarian) every so often (more on semivegetarian eating later).

DO VEGETARIANS GET ENOUGH PROTEIN?

A diet that uses no animal products lacks animal proteins, which normally supply large amounts of essential amino acids. Plant products (grains, beans, nuts, seeds, and vegetables) can supply these amino acids, but not by themselves. Ideally, they should be used in various combinations to complement the profile of amino acids found in each food.

To get complete protein from plants, you must combine legumes with grains or seeds. The principal source of protein for total vegetarians is usually a combination of grains and legumes. For example, a square of corn bread topped with a cup of cooked pinto beans provides the same amount of good-quality protein as two ounces of cooked lean beef.

Complementary protein foods should be eaten at the same meal. It's okay to eat an occasional meal of incomplete protein, as long as you eat the complementary protein a few hours later or at the next meal. Eating ½ cup of cooked beans (legumes) along with approximately 1⅓ cups of cooked grain will provide the essential amino acids in the proper proportions.

If you eat milk products (yogurt, cheeses), eggs, fish, or poultry, you get plenty of good-quality protein and needn't worry about combining plant proteins at each meal. Simple combinations such as milk poured over grain cereal or plain yogurt mixed in a pasta casserole provide balanced protein.

CALORIE CONCERNS:
DO VEGETARIANS HAVE STAMINA?

Just as important as the protein quality of a vegetarian diet is the number of calories it contains, especially for heavy exercisers. A totally vegetarian diet is higher in bulk than one containing meat—you simply eat more food. If you need 3,000-plus calories a day, salads just don't make it. Try eating more whole-grain cereals and breads, beans, nuts, and seeds. Eating peanut butter and crackers, for example, is a good way to get some protein and a heavy dose of calories.

However, you can easily get an overdose of calories and fat on a lacto-ovo vegetarian diet by lavishly using cheeses, eggs, and milk. Additionally, watch out for animal fats added to processed foods. (Select packaged foods with labels showing U or K, which are kosher symbols indicating no animal fats.) Select low- or nonfat dairy products to keep fat levels down. For instance, try nonfat yogurt on baked potatoes or low-fat cheese on a pizza. Add egg whites to dishes requiring whole eggs as a way to cut back on unwanted cholesterol.

DO VEGETARIANS FALL SHORT
ON VITAMINS AND MINERALS?

If you give up all animal products, you must eat certain foods or fortified foods to get specific vitamins and minerals.

Vitamin B_{12}. This vitamin is found only in animal products, so if you are a strict vegetarian, you must use vitamin B_{12}-fortified foods, such as soy milk, or take a supplement. Lacto-ovo vegetarians get sufficient amounts of B_{12} from milk or eggs.

Vitamin D. Here is another nutrient found exclusively in animal products. However, your body can make its own vitamin D even when only your hands and face are exposed to sunlight for 15 to 30 minutes daily.

Calcium and riboflavin. Intake of these may be inadequate if you don't use dairy products. But you will be fine if you get plenty of dark-green vegetables, legumes (particularly in tofu made with calcium carbonate), nuts, and seeds.

Iron. Lesser amounts of this mineral are present in vegetable sources—and are absorbed less efficiently—than iron from meats. Vegetarians, especially women, must be sure to eat foods that are good iron sources, including whole or enriched grains (like iron-fortified cereal), legumes, dried fruits, and green leafy vegetables (broccoli, turnip greens, kale, collards) that are low in oxalic acid, which keeps iron from getting into your bloodstream. If you include a vitamin C source at meals, you increase your ability to absorb iron.

Zinc. Levels of zinc can be marginal in vegetarian diets, since meats are the major source of zinc for most of us. Moreover, a high-fiber diet (from eating all those vegetables) will bind some of the dietary zinc and prevent its being absorbed by your body. What to do? Include regular servings of wheat germ, whole grains, and dried yeast to boost your zinc intake.

VEGETARIAN EATING MADE EASY

Many people shy away from eating as a vegetarian, with the thought that boiling beans and steaming rice takes time. It does, but like meals with meat, vegetarian dishes can also be made simply and quickly. Here are some tips to save time and take the hassle out of vegetarian cuisine. Whether you are already a vegetarian of sorts or are just looking for the health benefits from a few vegetarian meals added to your menu, my tips will save time.

Use quick-fix beans as a substitute for meat. Precooked canned kidney, fava, pinto, and garbanzo beans can easily be added to vegetable soups, stews, salads, and casseroles in place of beef, chicken, or other meats. Don't forget to combine with a grain product to make a complete protein.

Use whole-grain products when possible for added nutrients. Try quick-cooking instant brown rice, whole-grain pasta, and breads. Order whole-wheat pizza crust at your favorite pizza parlor and request wheat bread at restaurants.

Try meat substitutes made from soybeans. Usually in the freezer section of health food stores, these products are made to look like meat and can be prepared as meat is in only a few microwave minutes.

Use ready-made vegetarian products as time-savers. Items like veggie-burgers, meatless tacos, enchiladas made with tofu, and legume-stuffed ravioli and lasagna, found in health food stores and some supermarkets, are quickly prepared. But read

VEGETARIAN MENU

Here's a day's worth of easy-to-prepare lacto-vegetarian eating that has ample protein and lots of carbohydrates for stamina.

Breakfast

1½ cups whole-grain cereal with 1 cup low-fat milk and ½ cup strawberries

1 bran muffin with 1 teaspoon margarine

Lunch

Sandwich: two slices whole-wheat bread, veggie patty (tofu, carrots, zucchini, and onions), sprouts, and tomato slices

1 orange

½ cup raisins mixed with ¼ cup nuts

Snack

Blender drink: 1 banana, ¼ cup skim milk powder, ½ cup pineapple juice, and ice

Dinner

Three tortillas with 1 cup refried beans and salsa topping

Large green salad with 1 tablespoon oil-and-vinegar dressing

1 cup frozen yogurt

Analysis

Total calories: 2,550. Distribution: 65 percent carbohydrate, 15 percent protein (total protein: 90 grams), and 20 percent fat.

labels to make sure fat content is reasonable.

If you're omitting eggs, use ¼ cup tofu, one banana, or two tablespoons cornstarch as a substitute for each egg. Mix any one of these into a recipe as you would eggs.

Stick to ethnic restaurants when fast-food dining. Mexican fast-food restaurants offer bean and tortilla combinations with and without cheese, depending upon your preference. Chinese take-out dishes like tofu/vegetable combinations with plenty of steamed rice are quick, low-fat vegetarian meals.

Use meatless canned soups or sauces as a meal starter.
Simply add tofu chunks or canned beans and cooked rice or
another grain. Serve along with a salad or steamed vegetable,
and you have a quick-to-fix complete meal.

**Try packaged vegetarian chili mix or boxed rice dishes
for a main dish.** There are many "tofu-helper" type products
that require little time and few additions (canned beans or tofu),
and you can find these items in health food stores or in the health
food section of your local grocery store.

NEW VEGETARIAN DIETS

For an increasing number of people, vegetarian eating doesn't
mean going entirely meatless. Athletes are adopting the "new"
vegetarian eating style, which falls somewhere between the good
old American meat-and-potatoes routine and strict vegetarian
cuisine. Eating red meat, poultry, or fish just once or twice a
week (or less) is an eating style that many active people comfort-
ably opt for to cut back on fats and boost carbohydrates. Are any
body-refurbishing nutrients missing with this meat-sparse diet?
Or is it simply a ticket to better health and improved performance?

ALMOST *MEATLESS STYLE*

With the advent of worries over saturated fat and cholesterol,
many people, particularly athletes, began to dodge meat in their
diets. I work with many individuals who omit meat altogether,
adopting typical vegetarian fare of beans and rice and feeling
quite comfortable with their eating style. I've also noticed that
an increasing number of athletes and executives who attempt
meatless eating regimens gradually ease into a modified vegetarian eating style that includes weekly or biweekly use of animal
proteins.

This "new" vegetarian diet appears to represent a compromise
of sorts. True vegetarian eating requires more planning and extra
time to prepare traditional foods like combinations of whole
grains and cooked beans. Yet with our hectic not-a-minute-to-
spare lifestyle, we tend to rely on convenience foods and shy
away from anything that can't be microwaved within four minutes. I have also noticed that a great many of the "new" vegetari-

ans find a sense of nutritional security by occasionally eating meat of some sort. Surprisingly, many athletes and business types also tell me they simply crave meat every so often, and that's when they eat it.

Regarding this "new" vegetarianism, there are no set rules, as there are for strict vegetarians who eat no animal products (meats, eggs, or milk), or lacto-ovo vegetarians and lacto vegetarians who include eggs and dairy products or just dairy products. I find that each person approaches eating meats, eggs, and dairy products somewhat differently, modifying his menus for reasons of convenience, time constraints, and cravings rather than adopting a regular routine, such as eating chicken once a week and milk every other day.

A WORD OF CAUTION

I'll show how to avoid the problem of erratic and inconsistent meal planning, common among "new" vegetarians. The omission of meats, eggs, and dairy products should be met with the use of grains, beans, soy milk, and the frequent use of green leafy vegetables. These latter foods are sources of either protein, B vitamins, iron, or calcium left deficient by the exclusion of animal products. However, many individuals who sporadically eat meat and who have cut back on their use of dairy products and eggs seem not to be substituting traditional vegetarian staples to fill the nutrient void.

For example, among a group of dedicated endurance athletes I spoke with recently, over 50 percent ate meat less than once a week and dairy products less than once a day, yet few of them had replaced meat and milk with beans and whole grains, or increased vegetarian calcium or iron food sources. If you eat cereal without the milk and your dinners consist of salad, vegetables, and pasta without the meat, you should be adding complementary protein, like cooked beans or tofu.

This is the type of haphazard modified eating that may contribute to some of the ill effects seen with vegetarianism. Poor iron status, menstrual irregularities, and weaker bones are possible consequences when uncommon diets are not carefully thought-out.

A study from Ball State University in Muncie, Indiana, suggests that women runners who eat a modified vegetarian diet (less than four ounces of red meat a week) have iron-poor blood. Researchers matched runners who ate meat regularly with modified-vegetarian runners who had identical fitness levels, weekly training regimens, and dietary iron intakes. Despite an iron intake in both groups of just over two-thirds the RDA, the regular meat users had higher body iron stores and a healthier blood level of total iron binding capacity, indicating better iron status than the runners who ate meat no more than once a week.

Since iron from vegetable foods is less easily absorbed by the body than iron from red meats, fish, and poultry, these results suggest that attention to eating more iron-rich food sources is necessary when on a meat-sparse diet. Dried fruits, whole grains, cooked beans, and dark-green vegetables, for instance, are good iron sources that, along with vitamin C-rich foods (citrus fruits, tomatoes, green peppers, melons), improve iron's absorption by the body.

Further, high amounts of dietary fiber (typical in modified vegetarian diets that include mostly vegetable salads, grains, and bran cereals) may be linked to menstrual irregularity (including cessation of menses—amenorrhea) in women athletes. Athletes with menstrual irregularities consumed more fiber than did those with regular periods. (Both groups exercised equally and weighed the same.) Researchers suggest that high fiber intake, common in vegetarian diets, decreases circulating estrogen levels necessary for regular menstrual cycles. Estrogen is also important for maintenance of bone mineral density, which may help to explain the poor bone mineral content seen in many women athletes with amenorrhea.

Since "new" vegetarian diets appear to be a recent consequence of the 1980s cholesterol scare, their health benefits are not yet clear. Diets low in meats, eggs, and dairy products can certainly be a healthful change for athletes if they follow a few basic guidelines for avoiding nutritional mishaps. Just remember that a diet that includes very little meat is not necessarily better for you than a diet that includes meat regularly. Some vegetarian diets can easily contain more fat than a conventional meat diet does because of heavy use of cheeses, peanut butter, and vegetable oils.

BASIC GUIDELINES

You should be aware of any potential nutritional costs if you presently eat a modified vegetarian diet or plan to cut back on your use of meats, dairy products, and eggs. By selecting the right foods and learning how to combine them, you can avoid nutritional inadequacies that might sap your performance. Here are some solutions to common problems when planning your semivegetarian diet.

Problem: Red meat, fish, or poultry only once or twice a week will leave you short on meeting your protein needs.

Solution: On a daily basis, eat dried beans and grain combinations for quality protein. Canned vegetarian refried beans and quick-cooking brown rice, or tofu mixed into commercial nonmeat spaghetti sauce served over pasta, are quick vegetarian sources of protein and plenty of carbohydrates.

Problem: Substituting cheeses for meats can quickly boost the fat calories.

Solution: Use low-fat cheeses, like hoop cheese, part-skim or skim mozzarella, and dry-curd cottage cheese; keep serving sizes moderate—one to two ounces.

Problem: Lowered regular use of dairy products leaves you low on calcium.

Solution: Dark-green leafy vegetables, used in salads or quick-steamed for a side dish, provide a good source of calcium—as do tofu and calcium-fortified soy products.

Problem: Sparse meat consumption puts iron and zinc intake at a low.

Solution: Since these minerals are more available to the body from meats, make a special effort to eat good nonmeat sources regularly. Whole grains (refined grains are not enriched with zinc) and a variety of beans, including lentils, mung beans, and kidney beans, are good sources of zinc. Enriched and whole-grain products (breads, cereals, pastas) are mainstay sources of iron, along with dried fruit, dark-green vegetables, and beans.

Problem: Irregular eating habits lead to erratic nutrient intake.

Solution: Plan your meals, even if you think about dinner only five minutes before you eat it. If you are not including meat on your plate, you need to make up the difference with a simple substitute, such as pinto beans and rice, baked beans and corn bread, or steamed tofu and Chinese noodles.

SUPPLEMENTING PROTEIN: PILLS AND POWDERS

There's no doubt you need protein daily—your health and performance would erode if you routinely fell short of eating what you need. But do you need a protein supplement?

Open any magazine for muscle builders and you see the pages festooned with protein promises—everything from bigger muscles to faster recovery from exercise. But claims for protein supplements don't stop with body builders. Turn to almost any health and fitness magazine and you see claims that protein and amino acid supplements help melt off fat, improve your mood, curb aging, help you fall asleep, and may even help cure herpes. Could all or any of these promises be true? And more important, how safe are protein and amino acid supplements?

Before I answer these questions, let's look at what protein and amino acid supplements are all about. You can purchase quite a variety of supplements: protein powders and tablets; amino acid pills that contain one, two, or more individual amino acids; dipeptide and tripeptide pills (two or three amino acids connected in a chain); specific combinations of amino acids designed to speed recovery from exercise or stimulate muscle growth; and finally, proteins and amino acids combined with other nutrients like vitamins and minerals.

Depending upon the product, these supplements contain protein or amino acids, or both; and they most likely contain a filler of sorts to make up the bulk of the tablet. If you glance at the label, you notice that the ingredients usually are typical protein foods you eat. The manufacturers usually take soy protein or milk protein (casein) and put it in powder form or press it into a tablet. Oftentimes the instructions recommend mixing the protein powder with a glass of milk—an excellent protein source in itself!

Some manufacturers claim that predigested protein is better than the kind you get in food, but there is no evidence that healthy people—athletes and executives alike—have any trouble digesting or absorbing ordinary protein from food. Also, many products contain "free-form" amino acids, with claims that these amino acids will get into your system faster. But again, your body quickly digests all food protein into "free" amino acids. Also, your body does not recognize the difference between amino acids that originate from pills and amino acids that originate from foods.

Another point that deserves attention in the protein/amino acid supplement debate is how much protein a supplement provides and how this compares with what your diet contains. Depending upon the product, most protein powders supply 5 to 35 grams of protein (some of this coming from the milk it is mixed with). Check Table 3-3 for comparison—an average scoop of protein powder contains the same amount of protein found in two ounces of chicken or 1½ cups of beans and rice, with the same protein quality.

On the other hand, amino acid supplements, when compared with protein supplements, contain far less in the way of protein. Typical amino pills contain anywhere from 2 to 200 milligrams of amino acids. This is less than one gram. You get the same amount of amino acids from eating one ounce (two bites) of a good-quality protein, such as egg white, fish, chicken, or lean meat, at a fraction of the cost!

Protein Promises

Now let's turn to the claims made about protein supplements and their safety, particularly amino acid supplements, which are presently the most popular protein-type aid.

More muscle? Yes. But only if you're getting insufficient protein from your diet, which is unlikely. Earlier in this chapter I talked about how athletes need more protein—10 to 50 percent more. Strength athletes do seem to have bigger gains in strength and muscle size with an adequate protein diet (about 20 percent over the protein RDA). However, this extra protein is easily acquired by eating foods, and there is no evidence that the proteins from powders or amino acid supplements are superior to the proteins from milk, meat, or beans.

If taking a protein supplement is more appealing to you than eating extra rice and beans or grilled chicken, and if you do it in moderation, this practice is not harmful. The extra protein is not converted entirely to muscle. (Of an extra ten grams of protein from lean meat or a protein shake, little goes to muscle. A gain of over 30 pounds of new muscle a year would result from just this extra ten grams of daily protein, if it were utilized in this way.) I pointed out earlier that large protein intake presents health problems like calcium loss and dehydration.

Weight-loss aid? Claims that amino acids, taken singly or in special combinations, help with weight loss have been around for some time. Yet there is no scientific evidence to support these long-standing claims. Two amino acids, arginine and ornithine, are touted as able to "melt fat away while you sleep" by increasing the production of growth hormone. It's true that the same hormone that helps muscle size also controls fat metabolism. However, upsetting the hormone balance in your body to control fat metabolism would require massive amounts of these amino acids and would be debilitating and dangerous.

Since most amino acid supplements provide only a few milligrams per dose, their use would be impractical as a way to achieve the 1,500 milligrams of arginine required to spike the levels of growth hormone. And overproduction of this hormone can cause diabetes and acromegaly (a condition in which muscles enlarge but become weaker).

Other amino acids are said to aid in weight loss by suppressing the appetite. The amino acid phenylalanine, for example, has received much attention in this regard, since it is converted into norepinephrine, a brain chemical involved in appetite control. However, your body directly regulates how much norepinephrine it needs to make at any one time, so feeding on phenylalanine doesn't itself mean better appetite regulation.

It's fortunate that ingesting extra phenylalanine does not mean manufacturing more norepinephrine. This principle actually protects your body from going haywire whenever it is overloaded with specific building materials. For example, cholesterol is the building material for the male sex hormone, testosterone, but eating a half-dozen eggs or taking a cholesterol supplement does

POWER FOODS: THE FACTS

not cause an increase in the body's testosterone levels.

Faster recovery from exercise? There's no evidence that taking amino acids, either singly or in special combination, speeds up recovery from heavy exercise. There is plenty of evidence, however, that amino acids are broken down in your muscles for energy. The specific amino acids leucine, isoleucine, and valine (the branched-chain amino acids) are burned, just like carbohydrates, to help power your muscles during a long run or bicycle ride.

Despite this use of muscle protein, recovery from exercise is not improved with use of a branched-chain amino acid (BCAA) supplement. The spent amino acids are replaced from the ever-present pool of amino acids in the muscle tissue. This pool of amino acids is not influenced by popping a tablet or two of BCAA; rather, it is a product of your day-to-day diet and overall health.

Sleep aid? Yes. A number of scientific studies have shown that tryptophan, an essential amino acid, helps people with mild insomnia. There is also evidence that tryptophan may relieve some types of depression and chronic pain. This amino acid acts to aid sleep and improve mood by its conversion to the brain chemical, serotonin, which is involved in the sleep-wake cycle. The amount of tryptophan necessary to make you sleepy ranges from one to five grams.

Despite the potential sleep-inducing action of tryptophan, this amino acid, if taken in supplement form, can be deadly. A nationwide outbreak of over 1,400 cases (with more than 19 deaths) of eosinophilia—a sometimes fatal blood disorder characterized by severe muscle pain, weakness, fever, and skin rash—has been linked to the use of tryptophan supplements. In one case, a 58-year-old woman fell ill with eosinophilia and died three months later; she had been taking five to six grams of supplementary tryptophan daily. Subsequently, the FDA recommmended a nationwide recall and discontinued use of tryptophan products, typically sold in 500-milligram tablets.

A definite cause and effect has not been established between the use of tryptophan supplement and the disease, and health officials are also considering the possibility a contaminant in a particular brand or set of brands produced in Japan may be to blame. Foods normally provide about one to two grams of tryptophan each day, but because this dose is spread over the entire day, it has neither the same effect on hastening sleep nor any relationship to eosinophilia.

Anti-aging effect? Amino acids, such as cysteine, are said to help detoxify the body and curb the aging process by ridding the cells of potentially harmful toxins. There is no evidence to support such claims. Recent concerns about potentially harmful pollutants, chemicals in foods and the water supply that can cause cancer and speed up the aging process, have prompted many people to try such doubtful measures.

AMINO ACID SAFETY

Taking excessive doses of amino acids can be the potential cause of imbalances in amino acid levels in the bloodstream and, eventually, in the brain. We have little information about side effects of amino acid overdoses, but studies with animals do show that amino acid dosing causes problems with protein metabolism. While some amino acids show promise as a treatment for certain conditions, little is gained from taking these supplements specifically to achieve better performance.

IS MEAT OKAY?

M-E-A-T. It's a four-letter word to many health worshipers. During the past decade, we have cut down our consumption of red meat (beef, pork, lamb, and veal) to an average of about five ounces per person a day. Our intake of beef alone is down 20 percent. The fear of heart disease brought on by the fat and cholesterol content of meat, along with concern about meat additives and hormones, has turned many (particularly athletes) to a poultry and fish regimen, or even to a meatless lifestyle.

Still, many people are confused about meat. Some confidently eat it every day, while others, though they like red meat, feel guilty about eating it. Many are confused about whether giving up meat will result in losing strength or gaining health. You can simply and quickly answer your own to-eat-or-not-to-eat meat questions by knowing some basic facts.

PROS AND WOES OF MEAT

On the plus side, today's meats offer some outstanding nutritional values. Beef, pork, lamb, and veal are loaded with ready-to-use vitamins and minerals along with high-quality protein. Meats provide hard-to-get essentials like iron, zinc, vitamin B_6, and vitamin B_{12}. A three-ounce serving of regular ground beef, for example, provides you with the following part of your daily requirements: 50 percent of protein, 15 percent of iron, 33 percent of zinc, and 50 percent of vitamin B_{12}. This same three-ounce serving of beef supplies the same amount of protein, iron, and zinc as six ounces of chicken or two cups of black-eyed peas (the peas contain no vitamin B_{12}).

Although loaded with key nutrients, this same amount of beef has the disadvantage of containing 76 milligrams of cholesterol and 9 grams of fat—39 percent of which is saturated fat, the kind that elevates blood cholesterol. But there is a simple way to reduce these negative effects of meat:

□ Avoid high-fat cuts.
□ Trim the visible fat before cooking.
□ Limit servings to two to three ounces.

Use Table 3-6 to guide your meat selections.

BEST BEEF CHOICES

To get beef with the lowest fat possible, you have to consider both the cut and grade of meat. Meat grades—Prime, Choice, and Select—reflect the tenderness of the meat, which is directly related to how much fat, or marbling, is present. Prime grade beef contains the most marbling (fat), Choice somewhat less, and Select the least. Ask for Select grade at your local supermarket, and use slow cooking methods such as stewing or use marinades like lemon juice, wine, or vinegar to help make the meat more tender.

Choose those cuts that come from the leanest parts of the animal—legs, shoulder, belly, and neck—the parts that get the most exercise. These areas correspond to meat cut from the shank (lower leg), round (upper back leg), flank (belly), and chuck (neck and shoulder). Fattier meat cuts include the rib, loin, and sirloin, which can often sport more than twice as much fat as the leaner regions.

Table 3-6 *MEAT MARKET*

Here's how red meats, poultry, and fish stack up in calories, protein, fat, cholesterol, and nutrients. Serving size is 3 ounces, cooked.

| Meat | Calories | Protein (g) | Fat (%) | Cholesterol (mg) | Nutrients (% of USRDA) | | | |
					Iron	Zinc	B₆	B₁₂
Beef, top round, lean	164	27	29	72	14	32	24	35
Chicken, white meat, no skin	150	26	23	73	5	7	26	5
Cod	89	19	7	47	2	3	12	15
Lamb chop, lean	157	24	36	67	10	31	12	85
Pork tenderloin, lean	142	25	26	80	7	17	18	8
Salmon	157	23	37	42	4	3	9	95
Turkey, dark meat, no skin	160	25	34	73	11	26	15	5
Veal roast	184	23	46	100	6	31	16	52

SOURCE: Adapted from J. A. T. Pennington, *Bowes and Church's Food Values of Portions Commonly Used*, 15th ed. (Philadelphia: J. B. Lippincott, 1989).

Supermarkets now routinely offer "quarter-inch trim" meat cuts. And you may be able to find a new type of meat cut—the "total trim product"—at your local meat counter. By separating individual muscles, virtually all the fat can be removed. Total trim products, although more expensive than other meats, are sold in small portions to help control serving sizes.

HORMONE FEARS

Beyond worries about fat and cholesterol in meat, consumers fret over what they can't see or taste in meat—hormones and other growth stimulants. Worries range from cancer to early menstruation due to consumption of meat from hormone-treated cattle.

The meat industry is fighting hard to convince consumers of meat's safety. The fact is, hormones are used in livestock to speed up muscle growth, save meat producers money, and actually produce leaner cuts of meat. Hormone residue does show up in meat, but when compared with naturally occurring estrogen levels in men and women, the amount is inconsequential.

Estrogen, typically used in cattle as a slow-release implant beneath the skin, is naturally present in the animal. The amount of estrogen in a three-ounce piece of meat must be measured in nanograms—billionths of a gram. Here's how hormone-treated meat compares with untreated meat: Three ounces of cooked beef from hormone-treated cattle contains 1.9 nanograms of estrogen, while three ounces of cooked beef from untreated cattle contains 1.2 nanograms of estrogen.

When consumed by a woman, these levels have no effect on total body estrogen, which is in the neighborhood of 400,000 nanograms. Or for that matter, a man, with 100,000 nanograms of total body estrogen, is also unaffected by eating a serving of hormone-treated meat. No known medical or physical effects have occurred from eating this minimal amount of hormone. You can, however, purchase hormone-free meat by mail order or in some specialty meat shops.

FOR THE HEALTH OF IT

When weighing the pros and cons of a "beefed-up" diet, you must also consider what role meat plays in the health of both vegetarians and meat eaters. Vegetarian populations have lower serum cholesterol, blood pressure, and body weights than meat eaters. This translates into a reduced risk of cardiovascular disease.

But a vegetarian diet does not guarantee good health. Some groups of non-meat-eaters reap few benefits by restricting red meat intake. Women who are strict vegetarians or who eat only fish and poultry do not necessarily show lower blood cholesterol levels for their efforts, but instead exhibit depressed iron stores. Subnormal iron stores can progress to iron-deficiency anemia and lead to chronic fatigue and performance problems.

Meat is an excellent source of iron. It contains heme iron, which the body absorbs more easily than the nonheme iron found in legumes and vegetables. Also, scientists are exploring a yet-to-be-identified "meat factor" which results in a greater iron absorption from all foods eaten with red meat.

This same absorption-enhancing effect has been shown for zinc—a mineral marginal or low in the diets of most people. When meat is added to a meal, the absorption of zinc goes up. This means that small amounts of beef or pork added to an otherwise vegetarian meal of beans and rice can significantly improve zinc absorption from the beans and rice.

Even though meat's nutritional value is commendable, it is not indispensable. Nutritionally adequate diets can be created without red meat. However, if for ethical, religious, or economic reasons you choose to steer away from red meat, you must regularly eat other foods rich in zinc, iron, vitamin B_{12}, and protein.

If you do choose to eat meat, you must consider it as part of the total diet. Five ounces of lean meat per day, when combined with a low-fat, low-cholesterol, high-fiber diet, satisfies the nutritional recommendations made by the Surgeon General, the American Heart Association, and other professional health organizations.

But Americans are not always able to keep their diet ideally balanced. For instance, consumers report that they are purchasing leaner cuts of fresh meat and trimming the visible fat. However, these same consumers are also eating more processed meats, such as sausages and cold cuts, which contain more fat, sodium, and additives. Many of these processed meats have astounding fat levels. Check Table 3-7 to see how your favorite sandwich filler compares with the All-American favorite, hamburger. Most luncheon meats and sausages are extremely high in fat and are uncommendable sources of protein, vitamins, and minerals.

"NEW" BEEF

On the other hand, as a result of growing demand for leanness and convenience, the meat industry is responding with new products. For example, meat producers are providing leaner cuts of beef, pork, and lamb through specially bred "low-fat" livestock. Steers may look the same, but they are now trimmer in terms of fat than cattle of ten years ago. Changes in diet, breeding, and genetic engineering are helping to produce less fatty meat, particularly beef.

Lean and Free Brand beef products, for example, boast 73 percent less fat, 31 percent fewer calories, and 15 percent less cholesterol than comparable cuts of regular beef. Another line of low-fat beef to look for is Golden Trim beef, which has the same amount of fat as skinless chicken and some fish.

Other new meat products emphasize convenience. Red meats are reappearing in the frozen dinner lineup, which is currently dominated by fish and chicken dishes. And while luncheon and other processed meats are not the most nutritious foods (they may contain as much as 90 percent fat calories), the emergence of some reduced-fat and low-sodium products is a sign of the times.

Microwave cuts are gaining popularity at the meat counter. And believe it or not, many stores will soon feature exotic meats like buffalo, deer, and water buffalo. These meats, along with other game meats, are lower in saturated fat than conventional red meats.

If you've been considering the addition of red meat to your diet, now is a good time to make the move. Of course, it's up to you: By following a few basic guidelines, you don't have to eat red meat to be nutritionally complete.

Table 3-7 LUNCH MEAT LINEUP

What's your favorite sandwich filler? See how cold cuts compare on calories, protein, fat, and cholesterol.

Meat	Portion	Calories	Protein (g)	Calories from Fat (%)	Cholesterol (mg)
Bologna					
Beef	1 slice	72	2.8	82	13
Turkey	1 slice	60	3.9	67	19
Chicken roll	1 slice	45	5.5	42	14
Corned beef	1 oz.	43	6.0	36	13
Frankfurters					
Beef	1	142	5.4	81	27
Chicken	1	116	5.8	68	45
Ham, lean	1 slice	37	5.5	34	13
Knockwurst	1 slice	209	8.1	81	39
Liverwurst	1 slice	59	2.5	78	28
Pastrami					
Beef	1 oz.	99	4.9	75	26
Turkey	1 oz.	33	5.4	33	17
Polish sausage	1 oz.	92	4.0	79	20
Salami, dry	1 oz.	57	3.2	73	15
Turkey roll	1 slice	42	5.1	43	15

SOURCE: Adapted from J. A. T. Penningtor, *Bowes and Church's Food Values of Portions Commonly Used*, 15th ed. (Philadelphia: J. B. Lippincott, 1989).

CHAPTER **4**

HIGH-PERFORMANCE FATS

Fats are greasy, fattening, and troublesome when eaten in excess. You like the rich taste but despise the way fats linger in your body—clogging arteries, boosting your risk for cancer, causing weight gain, and making your performance sluggish. But despite their bad reputation, fats are actually essential for your health.

In this chapter, I show you which fats are the right fats for staying healthy. You learn:

- ☐ How to balance good and bad fats.
- ☐ The true story about cholesterol and health.
- ☐ The way to measure how much fat is best for your health and performance.
- ☐ The best fats for cooking.
- ☐ What to watch for on food labels.
- ☐ Simple ways to figure the fat in your diet.
- ☐ The best high-fat foods to choose.

This chapter will prove to you that an optimal balance of fat in your diet is your key to success and a longer, healthier life.

MOVING THE FAT

Understanding how fat is handled by your body will give you the facts you need to make fats work for you and your health. Whether you've eaten omega-3-rich fish or creamy cheesecake, your body must digest and move the fat from these foods through

(continued on page 124)

IMPORTANT FACTS ABOUT FATS

There's good news for everyone concerned about the effects fats have on the system. Certain fats can help you live longer. You will see that knowing what type of fat is in the food you eat (and how your body handles that fat) is vital to understanding the fat/health connection.

Whether it occurs in food or on your body, fat is a combination of fatty acids and glycerol (the same slippery liquid used to make soaps and skin lotions). Three fatty acids plus one glycerol make up a fat molecule, or triglyceride, as it's called by scientists. This triglyceride feels greasy to the touch, and like grease, it won't dissolve in water. Not all fat is created equal, however. Some fats are solid, like butter or the fat you see on a piece of meat. Other fats are liquid or more slippery, like vegetable oils or the fat in fish.

Just as some fats look and feel different from others, so do they have different effects on your health. Some fats may bring on heart disease, stroke, or cancers; others help to keep you free from certain cancers, arthritis, and migraine headaches and actually add years to your life. The good and bad health effects of fats are due in part to the type of fatty acids attached to the glycerol that makes up the fat molecule.

(continued)

Fats—*Continued*

Meet the Fat Family

There are three types of fatty acids, and each has a different impact on your health.

Saturated fatty acids: The chemical structure of these fatty acids makes them solid at room temperature. Many of the fatty acids in the triglycerides found in butter, beef fat, coconut and palm oil, and hydrogenated vegetable oil contain saturated fatty acids. This type of fatty acid has been shown to raise the risk for heart disease and stroke by raising the level of blood cholesterol which can eventually clog the arteries.

Monounsaturated fatty acids: These resemble saturated fatty acids but have a slight modification that changes the way monos behave *on the table* and inside your body. They are liquid at room temperature and are the predominant fatty acids in olive oil and canola oil. The body responds more favorably to monounsaturates since these fatty acids don't elevate blood cholesterol levels. In fact, some research studies show monounsaturated fats can actually lower blood cholesterol, reducing the risk for heart disease.

Polyunsaturated fatty acids: These look much like monounsaturated fats but have a slightly different chemical structure that makes polyunsaturates behave a certain way, and that is both good and bad. Polys are the major fatty acids in vegetable oils such as safflower oil and corn oil. In general, polyunsaturated fats lower blood cholesterol levels. However, high amounts of these oils in the diet may carry a greater risk for certain types of cancer.

The Best of the Fats

Two particular polyunsaturated fatty acids—linoleic and linolenic—are essential to humans for healthy skin, normal growth and nerve function, and proper wound healing. Without these two fatty acids, serious problems with performance and health arise. But fortunately, most of

(continued)

Fats—*Continued*

us take in plenty of these good fats every day. Only young children, or others who are being fed special diets through tubes, run the risk of receiving too little of these essential fatty acids.

Another type of polyunsaturates—the omega-3's—deserves special attention. They occur primarily in fish fat and are in demand by health-seekers, especially those trying to lower their risk of heart disease. These fatty acids are liquid, even in very cold temperatures (that's why they can function well in cold-water fish and other marine life). Due to their special chemical arrangement, omega-3's lower blood-fat levels and, therefore, heart disease risk. These fats also help prevent the development of blood clots, which can severely restrict the flow of blood to the heart.

Omega-3's benefits go beyond heart health. Studies of certain cultures, such as the Eskimos, who regularly eat fish rich in omega-3's, show that these fatty acids have an anti-cancer effect, lower high blood pressure, and help soothe arthritis pain. Additionally, scientific studies suggest that omega-3 supplementation cuts down on the number and severity of migraines.

Eat at least one to two fish meals a week to gain the omega-3 benefits. Fish oil pills, though they are presented as an appealing alternative to cooked fish, are costly and may not offer the same benefits you get from eating the real thing. Concentrate on the fish that are richest in these fatty acids.

As you can see, the type of fat you eat certainly does have an impact on your overall health, on the way you feel, and ultimately on your performance. Seek out the foods that contain the highest percentages of the good fats. Remember that the fat in food is not a single type of fatty acid but rather a mix. Butter, for instance, contains predominantly saturated fatty acids and therefore is dubbed a saturated fat.

Table 4-1 *OMEGA-3 CONTENT OF FRESH FISH AND OTHER SEAFOOD*

When the choice is yours, pick the seafood richest in omega-3's. This list will help you go for the gold available in a market or on a menu. Serving size is 3½ ounces raw.

High (more than 1 g)	Medium (0.5 to 1.0 g)	Low (less than 0.5 g)
Anchovy	Bass	Catfish
Capelin	Bluefish	Clams
Carp	Eel	Cod
Dogfish	Hake	Crab
Herring	Halibut	Flounder
Mackerel	Oyster	Haddock
Sablefish	Pollock	Lobster
Salmon	Pompano	Perch
Sardines	Rainbow trout	Pike
Scad	Rock fish	Scallops
Sturgeon	Shark	Sea bass
Trout (lake)	Smelts	Shrimp
Tuna		Snapper
Whitefish		Sole
		Squid
		Swordfish

SOURCE: Adapted from Frank N. Hepburn et al., "Provisional tables on the content of omega-3 fatty acids and other fat components of selected foods," *Journal of The American Dietetic Association* 86 (1986): 788–93.

your system. This process of fat transport, like the fats themselves, is both good and bad. Fats provide you with health-giving essential fatty acids that must reach all the cells in your body. Yet, if your fat transport system tilts out of balance, you run the risk of heart disease and stroke. The fats you choose to eat affect this delicate balance.

From the moment you swallow food containing fat, your digestive tract treats it differently from carbs or protein. Remember, fat won't dissolve in water and most of your body is water, so you would expect that fat from food must be somehow altered to dissolve in your watery body. But you have a remarkable inborn system for moving fats, bypassing this problem of solubility. In your intestines, small spheres of fat (triglycerides) which are coated with protein eventually get into your blood circulation. These fat balls are called lipoproteins and look much like minute marbles. They flow through your bloodstream, dropping off fat to various tissues, such as muscles, and to fat depots.

CHOLESTEROL COMES INTO THE PICTURE

Cholesterol is part of this fat transport picture, too. Despite all its bad press, cholesterol is an essential part of every cell in your body and must be continuously supplied to cells in need. Your liver makes the most of the cholesterol you have, but you also ingest some in foods such as eggs, cheese, and meats. Only foods from animals contain cholesterol; fruits, vegetables, grains, and vegetable oils are all cholesterol free.

Whether it comes from eggs or is made by your body, cholesterol is transported by lipoproteins. Different types of these lipoproteins contain varying amounts of cholesterol. Low-density lipoproteins (LDLs) contain the most, while HDLs, or high-density lipoproteins, contain less and actually remove cholesterol from your body.

Once encapsulated in the lipoprotein, the cholesterol moves freely through the body and is then passed off for use by body cells. There its job is to monitor what goes in and out of each cell.

This is the way fat and cholesterol transport is supposed to work, but sometimes things go wrong. When levels of cholesterol in the blood climb above a desirable point, this essential substance can turn deadly. When cholesterol can't be passed off to cells as fast as it is being manufactured or digested, it tends to build up on the inside of your artery walls, clogging blood flow and consequently increasing the risk of a heart attack or stroke. The higher your level of total blood cholesterol (which is a measure of cholesterol in all types of lipoproteins), the

Table 4-2 *FAT LINEUP*

The oils and fats you use in cooking count when it comes to avoiding cancer, heart disease, and other threats to health. Stick to those high in the polyunsaturates and stay away from those high in the saturated fats. Use the list below as your guide.

Dietary Fat	Saturated (%)	Monoun-saturated (%)	Polyun-saturated (%)
Canola oil*	6	62	22
Safflower oil	10	13	77
Sunflower oil	11	20	69
Corn oil	13	25	61
Olive oil	14	77	8
Sesame oil	14	40	42
Soybean oil†	15	24	54
Peanut oil	18	49	33
Margarine, soft	19	49	30
Cottonseed oil	27	19	54
Chicken fat	31	47	21
Lard	41	47	11
Palm oil	50	40	10
Beef fat	52	44	3
Butter	66	30	2
Margarine, stick	80	14	16
Palm kernel oil	86	12	2
Coconut oil	92	6	2

SOURCE: *Composition of Foods: Fats and Oils,* Agriculture Handbook No. 8-4 (Washington, D.C.: U.S. Government Printing Office, 1979).

NOTE: Percentages may not add up to 100 due to small amounts of omega-3 fats.

+10% omega-3 fatty acids.
†+7% omega-3 fatty acids.

higher your risk of a heart attack. More important, however, is your level of LDLs. These lipoproteins present a greater risk if they are high, since they contain the most cholesterol, which may eventually be deposited inside your arteries.

There's more to this lipoprotein story. Unlike LDLs, HDLs are considered good for heart health, since they remove cholesterol from the body by way of the liver. Thus, high HDL levels are great. Studies show that women and people who exercise regularly have higher HDL levels than men and nonexercisers. A blood test that measures the different lipoproteins gives you the best picture on how you're doing in the cholesterol/heart-health connection. Table 4-3 shows the desirable levels of cholesterol and LDL to keep you in good health.

Remember, it is the type of fat you eat that affects blood cholesterol and heart health. While researchers aren't exactly sure why, *saturated fats cause LDL levels to go up—which is not good; monounsaturated fats cause LDL levels to go down and may even boost HDL levels—which is good. Polyunsaturated fats lower total cholesterol, but both LDL and HDL levels are pushed down—which is good and bad.* There's more to the diet and heart disease story later in this chapter. I will show you how and what to eat to keep the LDL/HDL balance in your favor.

Table 4-3 *WEIGHING THE RISKS*

Here is an evaluation of blood cholesterol and LDL levels (mg./100 cc) classified by heart disease risk.

Blood Fat	Risk Factor		
	Desirable	Borderline High Risk	High Risk
Cholesterol	Less than 200	200–240	More than 240
LDL	Less than 130	130–160	More than 160

SOURCE: National Heart, Lung, and Blood Institute, The National Cholesterol Education Program, Adult Treatment Panel, No. 88–2926 (Bethesda, Md.: National Institutes of Health, Nov. 1987).

For now, realize that the families of saturated, monounsaturated, and polyunsaturated fats all have an impact on your health. Managing the amount of fat you eat and the amount of each type in your diet will give your body the balance it needs for a longer life.

HOW MUCH FAT DO YOU NEED?

It's simple. You must eat some fat—the right fats—for top health, peak performance, and a long life. In your body, fat has immense responsibilities. Fat protects your body's organs from injury, helps vitamins and other fat-soluble substances to move through your body, serves as a building block for your sex hormones, and keeps your skin healthy. On top of this, fat is a major source of energy while you sleep, sit, read, and do other light activities. So how much fat do you need to do all this?

You can stay in top form with surprisingly little fat in your diet. You only need those essential fatty acids that your body can't make—equivalent to about a teaspoon of corn oil daily. However, no one I've ever known eats only this amount of fat. Instead, people eat too much fat—averaging over 20 teaspoons daily of fat, most of it saturated. In fact, about 37 to 40 percent of the total calories Americans consume come from fat in their diet, while the optimal level is 25 to 30 percent of the total calories.

Eating about 25 percent your total calories as fat is ideal for performance and health. At this level, you give your body more than enough fat to stay healthy, but not enough to jeopardize your health. And you have room for performance-boosting carbohydrates. Besides total fat level in your diet, you need to consider the type of fat you're eating. The following three-way distribution will provide the balance you need for top health, as recommended by the American Heart Association and other professional health organizations.

□ Ten percent of total calories as monounsaturated fats, such as olive and canola oils

□ Ten percent or less of total calories as polyunsaturated fats, for example, corn, safflower, and sunflower oils

□ Less than 10 percent of total calories as saturated fats, which include coconut oil, lard, butter, and palm kernel oil

HOW TO FIGURE YOUR FAT INTAKE

With this information, you can determine how much fat is right for you. Aim for 25 percent of your total calorie intake as fat. For instance, if you take in about 2,400 calories daily, 25 percent or one-quarter of this would come from fats such as margarine; fat in meat, milk, and cheese; ice cream; and other fat-containing foods (2,400 calories times 0.25 (25%) equals 600 calories from fat).

Convert this 600 fat calories into grams of fat. Knowing that fat contains 9 calories per gram, divide 600 calories by 9 calories per gram to get fat grams (600 calories divided by 9 calories/gram of fat equals 67 grams of fat).

To get your personal fat number, you simply need to:

1. Estimate how many calories you take in daily (for details, check chapter 7).
2. Multiply this number by 0.25 to get fat calories.
3. Divide fat calories by 9 to get grams of fat.

Check Table 4-4 for a quick estimate of how much fat is best for you.

Table 4-4 *DISCOVER YOUR IDEAL FAT INTAKE*

Daily Calorie Intake	Grams of Fat at 25% of Total Calorie Intake
1,200	33
1,400	39
1,600	44
1,800	50
2,000	56
2,200	61
2,400	67
2,600	72
2,800	78

Table 4-5 *FAT FOODS*

Here's a brief list of common foods that pack a dose of fat. Add up the number of grams of fat for items you eat daily: Are you over your fat-gram number?

Food	Portion	Fat (g)
Pizza, cheese and pepperoni	2 slices	36
Ice cream, Häagen-Dazs	1 cup	34
Breakfast sandwich, fast-food type, egg and sausage	1	33
Fried chicken	1 thigh, 1 drumstick	25
Hamburger	¼ lb.	24
Cheesecake	2 in. slice	22
Corned beef sandwich	3 oz. meat, 1 tsp. mayonnaise	21
Hot dogs	2	18
Milkshake, fast-food type	11 oz.	17
Chocolate chip cookies	4	14
Hamburger, fast-food type	1 small	11
French fries	Regular	12
Bagel w/cream cheese	1 (1 oz. cheese)	10
Whole milk	1 cup	8

SOURCE: Adapted from J. A. T. Pennington, *Bowes and Church's Food Values of Portions Commonly Used,* 15th ed. (Philadelphia: J. B. Lippincott, 1989).

As you probably know, fat deficiency is not likely to be a problem for you. In fact, you can easily exceed your daily allotment of fat grams with a fast-food breakfast sandwich and standard burger lunch. Look at Table 4-5 to estimate how much fat you take in during a typical day.

ADD PERFORMANCE YEARS TO YOUR LIFE

Before I tell you how to get the fat you need and how to avoid the fats you don't want, I must tell you the truth, the whole truth, and nothing but the truth about fat and your health. As you know, fat is both good and bad for you. Yet many Americans are running scared from fat—not sure which is the best margarine to spread on their bread or which salad oil will help save their heart.

While I believe wholeheartedly that excessive fat is bad for you, much of the bad-fat/good-fat business has been overdone. It's important to consider the facts about dietary fats as they relate to heart disease and cancer and to realize that eating sensibly can add years to your life. But although diet plays a key role in your health, your lifestyle and exercise habits, the amount of rest and relaxation you get, and even your heredity also influence the length and quality of your life.

HEART DISEASE AND CHOLESTEROL

Whether you exercise regularly or not, you face the risk of a heart attack or stroke caused by the buildup of fatty cholesterol deposits in your arteries. Half of all deaths in the United States each year are caused by this blockage of arteries. But the true cause of the buildup of fatty deposits is under hot debate. Lately, most people single out diet, particularly fat and cholesterol intake, as the main culprit. Indeed, scientific evidence does link fat and cholesterol intake to heart disease, but these two "substances" are not solely to blame.

Other factors that increase your risk of developing heart disease include: high blood pressure (which with cholesterol is the major heart disease risk element); smoking; family history of heart disease; a sedentary lifestyle; age; gender (heart disease is more common in men); diabetes; low HDL levels; diet (low fiber intake, for example); and possibly behavior. All these influences, along with fat and cholesterol intake, figure into your equation for heart disease risk.

Many studies do show that a fatty diet—40 percent or more of the total calories—puts people at greater risk for a heart attack. But lowering fat in your diet will not necessarily free you from the risk of heart disease. The connection between fat in the diet and heart disease is blood cholesterol level. High blood cholesterol level is associated with a greater risk for heart disease. Thus, if you lower your cholesterol level, your risk for heart disease should be lower. But it isn't that simple, and that's where the case for drastically changing your diet to lower your blood cholesterol level comes under fire.

It's true. Scientific studies do show that blood cholesterol levels can be lowered in most people with dietary changes, such as cutting down on total fat or saturated fat intake. But these studies are done under tightly controlled conditions, quite different from those that surround you and me in the real world. Thus, spreading a margarine low in saturated fat on your bread or dressing your salad with olive oil might not actually cut *your* blood cholesterol levels or heart disease risk, as it might under laboratory conditions.

The best evidence to support the benefit of reducing fat and possibly cholesterol intake comes from studies involving middle-aged men with high blood cholesterol levels. These individuals appear to respond favorably by lowering their risk for heart attack with a drop in blood cholesterol. But for people who have desirable cholesterol levels (see Table 4-3), a low-fat diet may not further improve their chances against heart disease.

The case for cutting back on cholesterol in your diet is also weak. Your body makes cholesterol on its own, producing each day about four to five times the amount contained in one egg. But your body slows down cholesterol production when you eat more cholesterol and speeds up cholesterol production when you eat less of it. In fact, your body is geared by nature to control blood cholesterol levels.

However, not everything in nature always works as planned. Some people's systems don't regulate production very well, and their blood cholesterol level goes up when they consume excess cholesterol. These people may benefit from controlling dietary cholesterol, limiting intake to less than 300 milligrams daily (the amount in one egg and three ounces of lean beef). But be aware that many studies show no change in blood cholesterol levels for some people, no matter how much cholesterol they consume.

So paring down the excess cholesterol in your diet may not lower your own blood cholesterol levels at all and may result in a shortage of key nutrients if you're not careful. Many foods that contain cholesterol, such as eggs, meats, chicken, fish, cheese, and other dairy products, are great sources of essential power nutrients, such as protein, iron, zinc, and B vitamins, that you need to get from somewhere. For most people, moderate consumption of eggs and other cholesterol-containing foods poses no threat to blood cholesterol levels and heart disease risk. Check Table 4-6 for quick reference on the amount of cholesterol in some common foods.

Other dietary factors are linked to heart disease and must be considered along with fats and cholesterol. Fiber, for instance, lowers blood cholesterol. Water-soluble fiber (about 10 grams daily), of the type found in oats, psyllium seed, beans, and fruit, can help to lower blood cholesterol by as much as 15 percent. By binding with cholesterol in the intestinal tract, the fiber traps the unwanted cholesterol before it enters the body. Check Table 4-7 for top water-soluble fiber foods.

Besides fiber, you might want to consider your intake of garlic and onions, both known to have positive effects on blood-fat levels. Additionally, excessive caffeine intake or a low intake of the minerals magnesium and selenium may put you at higher risk for heart disease. When you stand back and look at the whole diet/heart disease picture, it's easy to get confused.

People tend to overemphasize specific dietary issues, like avoiding eggs at all cost or using olive oil in everything. I suggest you keep in mind the balance of carbohydrates, protein, and fat you need in your diet. Eating a diet that consists of 60 percent carbohydrate calories, 15 percent protein calories, and 25 percent fat calories will provide what you need for a healthy heart and lasting performance.

CANCER

Cancer also has strong roots in diet, particularly fat intake. But as with heart disease, dietary factors are not the sole cause for cancer. Lifestyle, heredity, and exercise habits, for instance, also play a major role in cancer. An estimated 30 to 50 percent of all cancer cases are linked to diet. Of these, a major number

Table 4-6 *CHOLESTEROL WATCH*

Here's the cholesterol content of some common foods. It's prudent to limit yourself to less than 300 milligrams of cholesterol daily.

Food	Portion	Cholesterol (mg)
Meat, Poultry, Fish		
Beef liver, cooked	3 oz.	335
Veal roast, cooked	3 oz.	100
Pork, cooked	3 oz.	80
Beef, lean, cooked	3 oz.	72
Chicken, no skin, cooked	3 oz.	73
Tuna, cooked	3 oz.	40
Dairy Products		
Egg	1 large	225
Ice cream, premium brand	1 cup	80
Cheddar cheese	1 oz.	30
Ice cream, regular	1 cup	20
Milk, 2% fat	8 oz.	18
Cottage cheese, low-fat	1 cup	10
Milk, skim	8 oz.	4
Fast Foods		
Egg McMuffin	1	259
McD.L.T.	1	110
Taco Bell taco salad	1	100
Kentucky Fried Chicken	1 breast piece	93
Chocolate shake	1	30
Taco Bell taco	1	21
French fries	Regular	9

SOURCE: Adapted from J. A. T. Pennington, *Bowes and Church's Food Values of Portions Commonly Used,* 15th ed. (Philadelphia: J. B. Lippincott, 1989).

of deaths occur from colon, uterine, and breast cancer, all of which are connected to excessive dietary fat intake.

Countries that have a low fat intake—less than 30 percent of the calories consumed—have a lower incidence of several types of cancer. Additionally, high intake of polyunsaturated fats (the same fats that lower blood cholesterol) is associated with certain types of cancer. The National Cancer Institute recommends a diet low in fat (30 percent or less of the calories consumed) and high in carbohydrate, with plenty of grains, fruits, and vegetables, to combat the threat of cancer. Besides lowering fat intake, this anti-cancer diet is high in fiber and rich in vitamins A and C and the mineral selenium, all of which have a protective effect against cancer. (More on these life-extending nutrients in the next chapter.)

THE POWER DIET SOLUTION

As you can see, the same paradox is apparent with the diet-cancer connection as with diet and heart disease. No one dietary

Table 4-7 *SOLUBLE FIBER*

Eat these foods frequently to get plenty of cholesterol-lowering fiber.

Food	Portion	Soluble Fiber (g)
Prunes	3	4.2
Heartwise cereal	1 oz.	3.0
Oat bran	1 oz.	2.0
Raisins	¼ cup	2.0
Kidney beans	½ cup	1.5
Oatmeal	1 oz.	1.4
Carrot	1	1.2
Apple	1 medium	1.0

SOURCE: Adapted from J. W. Anderson and S. R. Bridges, "Dietary Fiber Content of Selected Foods," *American Journal of Clinical Nutrition* 47 (1988): 440–47.

constituent can be cited as the cause of, or preventive against, cancer. Your best assurance for a long life free of cancer is to strike a balance in your diet, focusing your efforts on high performance meals and snacks. I can't emphasize enough the magic behind the ideal distribution of calories. Here is my 60-15-25 Power Diet—60 percent carbohydrate, 15 percent protein, and 25 percent fat.

I frequently tell people to stop worrying about what's bad for their health and start thinking about what's best for their performance. I'm convinced you will perform your best at work or during a workout—and live a healthier and longer life—by using my Power Diet.

STRATEGIES FOR CONQUERING THE FAT ISSUE

Now, how do you go about eating the fat you want and avoiding the fat you don't need? My simple strategies that follow give you the know-how to eat confidently, without fearing fat. Additionally, I give you the tools to make fat work for you—gaining from its health benefits and avoiding the kinds of fat that can sap your daily and lifelong performance.

You have two tasks at hand if you are to master the fat issue: Reduce your present fat intake to 25 percent of your total calories; and make lasting changes in your eating habits, food choices, and methods of meal preparation to keep foods convenient, tasty, and high-performance.

You won't have to disappoint your taste buds or hamper your schedule to eat a low-fat, high-performance menu. All it takes is a little fat-finding know-how to stay on the fast track in a tasty way.

For starters, know your *fat number*—the number of fat grams that provides 25 percent of your total calories as fat. Estimate your fat number based on your approximate calorie intake. You can also calculate the number using this formula:

1. *Calories/day* $\times$ *0.25* = *number of fat calories*

2. *Fat calories* $\div$ *9 calories/gram of fat* = *number of grams of fat daily*

Once you have your fat number, use it to guide your food choices at fast-food outlets, restaurants, grocery stores, and your workplace vending machines.

The next step is to divide your fat number by the number of meals and snacks you have daily. This will give you the number of fat grams to work with each time you eat, thereby sparing you from keeping track of fat grams all day long.

I'll use myself as an example to show you how easy fat gram counting can be: I average about 2,400 calories daily, of which 25 percent comes from fat. This translates into 67 grams of fat— my fat number (2,400 calories times 0.25 divided by 9 calories/ gram) is 67 grams. Typically, I eat five equal-sized meal/snacks each day, and this translates into approximately *13 grams of fat each time I have a meal* (67 grams of fat divided by five meals equals 13 grams of fat per meal).

Knowing this figure enables me to pick up packaged foods, look at the nutrition label, and decide if a particular food "blows" my fat budget. For instance, a TV dinner that packs 25 grams of fat takes up nearly two meals' worth of allotted fat (26 grams). For foods like cheese and meats that don't have a label, I use a list similar to the one in "Fat-by-the-Gram Listing" on page 138 to guide my food choices.

Knowing your fat number will get you started in the right direction toward achieving 25 percent fat calories and better performance. To keep you going in the right direction, I show you:

□ How to cut back on fat.
□ How to detect hidden fat in prepared foods.
□ The best ways to prepare and cook low-fat meals.
□ The best fats to use for eating and cooking.
□ Low-fat foods to substitute for high-fat favorites.

CUT THE FAT

Perhaps the best place to start working toward the 25 percent fat diet is take aim at the added fats in your diet—butter, margarine, mayonnaise, salad dressings, and cooking oils—since the majority of these foods are almost pure fat. These items can quickly push your fat intake over your fat number target.

For instance, one teaspoon of butter, margarine, or vegetable

FAT-BY-THE-GRAM LISTING

Here, foods are listed by category for quick reference of fat content. Use these numbers as a guide when making selections for a meal or doing your weekly shopping.

Breads, Cereals, Pasta, Grains

The following foods have little or no fat.

- Bagel
- Bread
- Cooked cereal
- Corn
- Lentils, kidney beans
- Pasta (not egg noodles or Ramen-type noodles)
- Potato
- Ready-to-eat cereal (except granola)
- Rice

Meat, Fish, Poultry

The following lean foods have 9 grams of fat per 3 ounces.

- Chicken, no skin
- Fish, most types
- Lean beef
- Lean pork
- Turkey, no skin
- Veal

The following regular foods have 15 to 24 grams of fat per 3 ounces.

- Most beef and pork cuts
- Chicken, with skin
- Hot dog and other sausage
- Lamb
- Luncheon meat
- Salmon
- Tuna in oil

Dairy Products

The following foods have no fat.

- Nonfat yogurt
- Skim milk

(continued)

Listing—*Continued*

Dairy Products

The following portions of low-fat foods have 5 grams of fat.

☐ 1 cup low-fat yogurt
☐ 1 ounce part-skim cheese
☐ 1 cup 2% milk

The following whole-milk foods have 8 grams of fat for the portions shown.

☐ 1 cup whole milk
☐ 1 ounce whole-milk cheese (cheddar, Swiss)
☐ 1 cup whole-milk plain yogurt

Fats and Oils

The following foods have 5 grams of fat for the portions shown.

☐ 6 whole almonds
☐ 1 slice bacon
☐ 1 teaspoon butter
☐ 1 teaspoon margarine
☐ 1 teaspoon mayonnaise
☐ 1 tablespoon salad dressing
☐ 2 whole walnuts

Fruits and Vegetables

All types of fruits and vegetables, whole and juice, have no fat, except for avocado, which has 20 grams of fat per half.

oil contains five grams of fat. Simply cutting back on the amount of butter or margarine you spread on bread or melt over vegetables and potatoes can easily save you five to ten grams of fat intake. Switching to reduced-calorie versions of margarine, mayonnaise, and salad dressings also pares down your fat intake. Most of these low-cal products lose little in flavor, so you won't feel cheated.

However, a word of caution is in order when you buy fat-modified products. Oftentimes a food label may boast that the food is cholesterol free. This *doesn't* mean that the food is lower in fat or calories. Cholesterol-free mayonnaise has calories and grams of fat equal to the cholesterol-containing version.

Be cautious about food labels that read "contains no tropical oils," meaning no coconut oil or palm oil. This does not mean the food is lower in fat but merely that another fat was used instead of the tropical oils. The product may still be high in saturated fat, depending upon what fat was used to replace the tropical oils. Read the nutrition label on the back of the package to check on how much fat the product contains.

Use Table 4-8 to see how much fat there is in your favorite salad dressing or margarine. Keep in mind that each gram of fat gives you nine calories, more than twice the four calories per gram that carbohydrates or protein contain.

FIND HIDDEN FAT

Look out for foods with "hidden" fat. Some foods that you would expect to be high in carbs or protein pack a surprising dose of fat. Snack crackers, for example, contain 30 to over 50 percent fat calories—this from a food you would think is mostly carbohydrate! Microwave popcorn, waffles, and various cookies are among the many common foods that contain hidden fat. (If it's crunchy, chances are good that the food has a considerable amount of fat.)

Many of these foods are packaged with a nutrition label that lists the number of fat grams per serving. Use this number and compare it with your daily fat number. If it is more than one-fifth of your daily fat allotment, that food is best left uneaten. For quick reference, you can also calculate the percent of fat calories in a food you're about to buy. All it takes is two simple steps:

1. Multiply the number of fat grams given on the nutrition label by 9 to get the number of fat calories.

2. Compare this number to the total number of calories per serving of food to get a percentage of fat calories.

For example, microwave popcorn has eight grams of fat per two-cup serving (115 calories). Here is how you calculate percentage of fat calories:

1. 8 grams × 9 calories/gram of fat = 72 fat calories.

2. 72 fat calories ÷ 115 calories/serving = 62 percent of calories from fat

Table 4-8 *FAT COUNTS FOR SPREADABLE AND POURABLE FATS AND OILS*

Fat or Oil	Portion	Calories	Fat (g)
Spreads			
Mayonnaise	1 Tbsp.	100	11
Cream cheese	1 oz.	100	10
Miracle Whip	1 Tbsp.	69	7
Butter	1 tsp.	36	5
Cream cheese, light	1 oz.	62	5
Margarine	1 tsp.	36	5
Margarine, whipped	1 tsp.	23	3
Mayonnaise, imitation	1 Tbsp.	35	3
Margarine, diet	1 tsp.	17	2
Regular Salad Dressings			
Ranch	1 Tbsp.	80	8
Italian	1 Tbsp.	69	7
French	1 Tbsp.	67	6
Thousand island	1 Tbsp.	59	6
Low-Calorie Salad Dressings			
Ranch	1 Tbsp.	40	4
Thousand island	1 Tbsp.	24	1.6
Italian	1 Tbsp.	16	1.5
French	1 Tbsp.	22	1

NOTE: Data derived from product labels.

Try to choose packaged food that contains no more than 30 percent fat calories. However, if a food is used as part of a meal that is otherwise very low in fat, then a higher percentage is acceptable.

Become familiar with foods that have hidden fat and try to choose them less often. Table 4-9 will help you be a fat-wise consumer.

Table 4-9 *HIDDEN FAT FOODS*

Don't let fat sneak into your diet. Be aware of these common fat traps.

Food	Portion	Fat (g)
Cheese omelet with 3 eggs	1	40
Chili and beans, canned	1 cup	23
Hostess snack pie	1	20
Coleslaw	½ cup	16
TV dinner	1	15–50
Croissant	1	12
Carrot cake	1 slice	11
Potato salad	½ cup	11
Muffin, bakery-type	1	10
Ramen-style noodles	1 cup	7
Sweet roll	1	7
Cream of tomato soup	1 cup	6
Granola bar	1	6
Frozen vegetables with sauce	½ cup	6
Biscuit	1	5
Ritz crackers	4	4

SOURCE: Adapted from J. A. T. Pennington, *Bowes and Church's Food Values of Portions Commonly Used,* 15th ed. (Philadelphia: J. B. Lippincott, 1989).

NOTE: Some data derived from product labels.

MAKE IT LOW-FAT

The ingredients and methods you use in preparing and cooking meals is another way that fat sneaks into your diet. The way you cook, toss a salad, make a sauce, or top a cake can greatly influence your daily fat intake. Additionally, with your fast-paced schedule, you probably don't have time to do much cooking from "scratch," so you're more apt to use ready-made ingredients that can add extra fat to your diet. For instance, packaged, dry pasta salads that require only boiling water and a little mixing are usually loaded with fat—over 40 percent fat calories.

The following strategies will help you in the kitchen, whether you're throwing a meal together in minutes or spending a few hours preparing a special meal.

Prepare food before cooking to lower fat content.

☐ Trim excess fat from meats.

☐ Remove skin from poultry.

☐ Skim fat off broth that is to be used in soups and sauces.

☐ Drain oil from canned meats and fish.

☐ Use water-packed tuna.

Use less fat when cooking.

☐ Use nonstick pans.

☐ Reduce the amount of butter or margarine used for sautéing or in recipes.

☐ Substitute nonfat dry milk for half the fat in a recipe for muffins, cookies, or quick breads.

☐ Use nonstick spray instead of added fat.

☐ Choose olive, canola, corn, safflower, or sunflower as cooking oils and use less.

Use low-fat cooking techniques.

☐ Steam or use the microwave for veggies.

☐ Broil, braise, or poach meats, chicken, or fish.

☐ Avoid frying foods of any kind.

Select lower-fat ingredients.

☐ Choose lean cuts of meat (round steak, sirloin, extralean ground beef).

☐ Try using spices, lemon juice, specialty vinegars, garlic and onion powder, or mustard in place of butter, cream, or mayonnaise.

☐ Read the label when buying packaged ingredients (for example, pasta salads) and apply the 30 percent rule.

☐ Use veggies to top a pizza instead of sausage or pepperoni.

☐ Substitute low-fat or nonfat yogurt for sour cream in casseroles or sauces.

☐ Substitute evaporated low-fat or skim milk for cream in sauces and desserts.

☐ Sprinkle Butter Buds or other imitation butter products on hot vegetables, baked potatoes, or air-popped popcorn.

☐ Choose jarred or fresh marinara pasta sauce over higher-fat meat sauces.

BEST FATS FOR COOKING AND EATING

When it's time to dress a salad or add margarine to a recipe, how do you know which is the best fat to use? Besides using less oil on your salad, you also want to choose an oil that's best for your health and your performance.

There are two considerations when choosing the best fat to use for cooking or eating. Select a fat low in saturated fat; select a fat high in monounsaturates.

From Table 4-2 (earlier in this chapter), you can get a good idea of which fats are low in saturated fats and high in monounsaturated fats. Canola oil, for instance, is the lowest in saturated fats, while olive oil is the highest in monounsaturated fats. Safflower oil and corn oil are good choices for avoiding saturated fats, and they are great sources for the essential polyunsaturated fatty acids.

When making your oil or margarine/butter selection, realize that they all contain the same number of calories per teaspoon. Oils labeled as "light," like olive oil and other cooking oils, are only lighter in taste or color—not in calories. "Light" olive oil, for example, has been filtered to remove the olive residue, giving the oil a lighter taste and color and making it great for baking. Diet margarines, however, do contain fewer calories per teaspoon or per ounce, since water is added during processing.

If you're watching cholesterol in your diet, remember that only fats from animal products contain cholesterol. Butter and lard are the animal fats most commonly used in cooking, and each contains about 11 milligrams cholesterol per teaspoon. Of more concern in these and similar fats is their high saturated fat content. Hard stick margarine is even higher in saturated fat than butter or lard, since it is made from hydrogenated vegetable oil—liquid vegetable oil (polyunsaturated) turned hard (saturated) by processing. To get through this bewildering minefield, follow the guidelines in "Be Smart about Fats" on page 148.

LOW-FAT SUBSTITUTIONS
FOR YOUR HIGH-FAT FAVORITES

As you've seen, there are many strategies you can use to balance your fat level at 25 percent of total calories. I suggest you try two or three different techniques every few days to get on track to a low-fat eating style. Table 4-10 lists easy-to-do substitutions that save you calories and fat and give your performance a boost at the same time.

REAL FAT, FAKE FAT, AND BODY FAT

Now you have a good idea of fat's significance in your day-to-day performance. Enough fat of the right type in your diet is crucial for good health, stamina, and a long life. If you eat too much fat, however, particularly the wrong type, your arteries become clogged, you face the threat of cancer, and you have a less-than-energetic way about you.

FAT IS DIFFERENT

But there's more to the fat story. Fat means fat. Compared with protein and carbohydrate, fat from the foods you eat is the most likely to end up as body fat. Simply put, one fat calorie is not the same as one carbohydrate or protein calorie. This difference in energy value between fat and carbohydrate and protein is contrary to what scientists thought a few years back. In those days, any nutritionist would have told you that a calorie is a calorie, regardless of its source. Since then, studies have shown that incoming food fat is handled preferentially by your body, ending up as body fat more readily than carbs and protein. In essence, one fat calorie is worth more than a carbohydrate or protein calorie.

As you discovered in chapter 2, for every 100 calories of extra fat you take in, 97 calories can be stored as fat, and the remaining 3 calories are burned for this storage process. But if you take in surplus calories as carbohydrate (e.g., pasta or sugar), your body does not convert the extra carbohydrate to fat very efficiently. Your body wastes about 23 calories out of every 100 carbohydrate calories just to convert the carb to fat. This means you put away only 77 calories as fat out of 100 extra calories eaten as carbohydrate.

Not only is it more expensive to convert extra carbohydrate calories to fat, your body seems very reluctant to do it. Studies with healthy volunteers show that large amounts of extra carbo-

Table 4-10 *MAKE THE SWITCH*

Try these simple substitutes for higher-fat foods for eating or cooking. You'll save big!

Instead of . . .	Choose . . .	And Save . . .
Snack Foods		
2 chocolate chip cookies	2 fig bars	30 calories
1 oz. potato chips	1 oz. pretzels	40 calories
2 cups microwave popcorn	2 cups air-popped popcorn	82 calories
10 oz. regular milkshake	10 oz. milkshake with ice milk and skim milk	100 calories
½ cup peanuts	½ cup dried fruit	300 calories
Meats		
3 oz. regular hamburger	3 oz. lean hamburger	65 calories
1 piece fried chicken	1 piece roasted chicken	75 calories
3 oz. oil-packed tuna	3 oz. water-packed tuna	90 calories
4 oz. fried fish fillet	4 oz. broiled fish fillet	120 calories
Dairy Products		
1 oz. cream cheese	1 oz. reduced-fat cream cheese	40 calories
8 oz. whole milk	8 oz. skim milk	70 calories
2 tsp. butter or margarine	1 serving Butter Buds	70 calories
2 oz. hard cheese (cheddar)	2 oz. part-skim cheese (mozzarella)	110 calories
½ cup sour cream	½ cup low-fat yogurt	240 calories
½ cup heavy cream	½ cup evaporated low-fat milk	250 calories

(continued)

Table 4-10—*Continued*

Instead of . . .	Choose . . .	And Save . . .
Miscellaneous		
2 slices pizza topped with meat	2 slices vegetarian pizza	80 calories
1 slice pound cake topped with whipped cream	1 slice angel food cake topped with low-cal whipped topping	80 calories
2 doughnuts and coffee with cream	1 cup whole-grain cereal with skim milk	180 calories
Fast-food fried chicken sandwich with vegetables	Fast-food baked potato stuffed with vegetables (no margarine)	125 calories
Fast-food hamburger and french fries	Fast-food salad with low-cal dressing	280 calories

SOURCE: Adapted from J. A. T. Pennington, *Bowes and Church's Food Values of Portions Commonly Used,* 15th ed. (Philadelphia: J. B. Lippincott, 1989).

NOTE: Some data derived from product labels.

hydrates must be eaten before fat conversion occurs. This doesn't mean carbohydrate calories don't count, but these re-sults do suggest you can eat more calories if your overall diet is low in fat and high in carbohydrate.

Another disadvantage to fat over carbohydrate: When you take in extra fat, your metabolism doesn't increase the use of fats for energy. Instead of revving up fat-burning activity, your body takes this extra fat and tucks it away in fat cells. On the other hand, when carbohydrates are eaten to excess, they actually step up your metabolic furnace. You use more carbohydrate for energy, so little of the extra pasta or potatoes has the chance to be converted to fat and put away in storage.

BE SMART ABOUT FATS

Here's a guide to healthful fat choices for cooking and eating.

☐ Substitute canola oil or "light" olive oil in recipes that call for melted butter, margarine, or vegetable oil.

☐ Use canola oil or regular olive oil for salad dressings.

☐ Use "light" olive oil instead of regular olive oil for stir-frying. (Regular olive oil smokes at high heat because of burning olive particles.)

☐ If you like the taste of butter for sautéing, use a small amount in the pan for flavor along with some canola, corn, sunflower, or safflower oil, or butter-flavored nonstick spray.

☐ Try olive oil as a flavorful alternative to margarine or butter on breads, bagels, or muffins.

☐ When buying margarine, choose brands with vegetable oil as the first ingredient on the label and check the label for low saturated fat content. Ideally, the margarine should contain twice as many grams of unsaturated as saturated fat.

☐ Use whipped margarine (usually in tubs) in place of regular stick-type margarine as a spread on breads or hot vegetables, for a savings of 30 calories or three grams of fat per tablespoon.

☐ Try diet margarine in place of regular margarine (except in baking, since it has a high water content which affects the recipe) for a savings of 40 to 60 calories per tablespoon (four to six grams of fat).

Fat's energy-efficient behavior helps explain why some people can't lose weight when they consume a low-calorie but relatively high-fat diet. In addition, researchers find that overweight people do not necessarily overeat, but they do eat a high-fat diet. This suggests obesity is linked to excess fat intake rather than to eating too many calories. A high-fat diet may also boost the desire to eat more food and the preference for fatty foods, only to aggravate the problem of obesity. Many overweight people choose higher-fat versions of foods like ice cream when given the choice.

In chapter 7, I provide more information concerning issues of weight control and fat intake, but for now, realize fat's powerful influence on you, your health, performance, and well-being. Researchers keep looking for solutions to the various health dilemmas that fats present. Artificial fats may be one way to lessen fat's catastrophic effects.

FAKE FATS

The fat substitutes, such as Olestra, from Procter & Gamble, and Simplesse, from NutraSweet, sound too good to be true. They promise to revolutionize eating and possibly to improve the nation's health. These products would replace conventional oils, shortenings, and butter in foods—effortlessly lowering calories, fat, and cholesterol intake.

Olestra, made from oil and sugar and processed into a synthetic molecule too big to digest, passes through the body unabsorbed. Procter & Gamble plans to use calorie-free Olestra as part of cooking oils, in deep-fat frying for fast foods, and in salted snacks. This means once-forbidden high-fat chips and baked goods might become a carbohydrate lover's delight—without guilt. However, foods made with Olestra will need to be fortified with vitamin E, since Olestra cuts the body's ability to absorb this fat-soluble vitamin.

Simplesse substitutes for fat in salad dressings, mayonnaise, butter spreads, ice cream, dips, and spreadable cheese products. Unlike Olestra, Simplesse is considered a natural food product and is digested and absorbed by the body, providing a fraction of the calories present in an equal amount of fat. Simplesse, which looks and feels like mayonnaise, is made from egg or milk protein that has been cooked and blended to form tiny balls that fool the tongue with fatlike slipperiness. Substituting cholesterol-free Simplesse for fats will greatly reduce fat calories while slightly increasing protein intake.

Depending upon how these fat substitutes are used, calorie savings could range from 40 to 80 percent. Using these fake fats in place of real ones will have a significant impact on our fat and cholesterol intake and possibly our health as well. Presently, we eat just under 40 percent of our calories from fat—well over the recommended intake. With the use of Simplesse and Olestra in a variety of foods, fat calories could be brought under the suggested 30 percent level and the average cholesterol intake brought closer to the 300-milligram daily limit.

Lowering fat intake with fake fats may also prove to be heart healthy. Blood cholesterol levels, along with body weight, were lowered to a greater extent in overweight subjects fed Olestra than in those fed the same low-calorie, low-cholesterol diet without Olestra. Researchers expect more in the way of health benefits from the use of fat substitutes—decreased risk of high blood pressure and of certain types of cancer may result from lower calorie and fat intake.

Table 4-11 *EXAMPLE OF CALORIE AND FAT SAVINGS WITH SIMPLESSE*

Product	Portion	Traditional		Made with Simplesse	
		Calories	Fat (g)	Calories	Fat (g)
Mayonnaise	1 Tbsp.	100	11	21	<1
Ranch-style salad dressing	1 Tbsp.	80	8	16	<1
Sour cream	1 Tbsp.	51	5	20	<1
Vanilla ice cream	4 oz.	274	19	120	<1

CHAPTER **5**

VITAMINS AND MINERALS:
too little or too much?

You can't see the vitamin C in an orange or the calcium in a glass of milk. For that matter, you can't see the vitamins or minerals in your body, but they are there, keeping you alive. Perhaps this mysterious or intangible nature of the vitamins and minerals helps explain why many of us fear that our diet is inadequate—bordering on vitamin or mineral deficiencies that can sap day-to-day performance. We convince ourselves that taking vitamin and mineral supplements will make up for what our food lacks or compensate for a missed meal.

Getting too little of any vitamins and minerals does sap your performance and compromise your health. You require a continual supply of these nutrients to feed your metabolism and rejuvenate your body's cells. But take in too much by misusing vitamin and mineral supplements, and you face a host of ills ranging from skin changes and hair loss . . . to death.

In this chapter, my guide "From A to Zinc" shows you how to find a balance between too little and too much. You also learn what the Recommended Dietary Allowances for vitamins and minerals really mean to you and whether this allotment is enough to meet your daily work and exercise demands. I highlight the standout vitamins and minerals for top health and give you the Top Ten Super Foods for vitamin and mineral nutrition. There's more—why you get fatigued, for example (you may need more iron for stamina), and the facts about the advantages and disadvantages of taking vitamin and mineral supplements.

FROM A TO ZINC

All told, a combination of 30 vitamins and minerals is required for good health. For the most part, your body can't make vitamins or minerals, so the food you select must supply these vital substances. The following is a brief overview of what these unique nutrients do for you and your performance.

MEET THE VITAMINS

From vitamin A on down to vitamin K, these nutrients in minute quantities facilitate hundreds of biochemical reactions in your body. Vitamins also act as regulators that oversee processes like bone growth and the maintenance of healthy skin. So important are the vitamins that, without them, you would be unable to process the carbohydrates you need for stamina, your body's protein metabolism would fall apart, and you would slowly degenerate—become anemic, weak, unable to think clearly, and, yes, eventually die.

Each of the 13 vitamins has specific functions. The B vitamin thiamin, for example, is vital for carbohydrate and energy metabolism. Vitamins are divided into two groups, based on their behavior in the body. The first group—the water-soluble vitamins, found in the watery parts of body cells—are vitamin C and the eight B vitamins (thiamin, riboflavin, niacin, B_6, pantothenic acid, B_{12}, biotin, and folate). These vitamins function as assistants in enzyme-driven chemical reactions. While they are key to energy metabolism, they do not provide energy by themselves.

The second group of vitamins—A, D, E, and K—are called fat-soluble, since they are found in the fatty parts of body cells. These vitamins act more as metabolic regulators. Vitamin A, for example, is responsible for keeping all of your mucus-lined tissue and skin healthy, while vitamin D is in charge of directing calcium into your bones. Check Table 5-1 for more on specific vitamin functions. As you can see, vitamins have many duties that all come together, keeping you healthy and performing your best.

VITAMINS IN FOOD

Virtually all foods, from carrots to chocolate-chip cookies, contain vitamins. Very small amounts, figured in milligrams or even micrograms (1/1,000,000 of a gram!), are present in a typical serving of food. But as you'll see in the next section, you only need very small amounts. A quick look at the table gives you an idea of the many different types of food that contain any one vitamin. As you can see, eating a variety of foods makes it possible to take in all the vitamins you need.

Despite this wide availability of vitamins, many of us fall short of our daily requirement due to poor food choices. In general, when whole foods like fruits, vegetables, and whole grains are processed in any way—peeled, cooked, separated—vitamin content is lowered. So for better vitamin nutrition, you should include unprocessed foods like fresh fruits and vegetables plus a variety of whole-grain breads and cereals in your daily diet.

Vitamins are also lost from foods when simple steps aren't taken to protect them. Aside from high temperatures and long cooking times, exposure to air, water, and even light can destroy certain vitamins in foods. For instance, when milk is stored in a glass container, light can have a negative effect on the milk's riboflavin. Also, if you slice vegetables and soak them in water, many of the water-soluble vitamins are likely to leach out, lowering the vitamin content.

Get the most vitamin nutrition out of the foods you eat by following these simple guidelines:

□ When preparing vegetables for cooking, cut them into larger pieces for better vitamin retention.

(continued on page 156)

Table 5-1 *VITAMINS: FROM A TO K*

Vitamin	Function	Food Sources
Vitamin A	Necessary for normal vision in dim light; maintains normal structure and functions of mucuous membranes; aids growth of bones, teeth, and skin	Yellow-orange vegetables and fruits, dark-green, leafy vegetables, fortified milk, eggs, liver
Thiamin (B_1)	Necessary for carbohydrate metabolism; helps maintain healthy nervous system	Pork, liver, whole-grain and enriched grain products, beans, nuts
Riboflavin (B_2)	Needed for protein, fat, and carbohydrate metabolism and healthy skin	Dairy products, whole-grain and enriched grain products
Niacin (B_3)	Needed for protein, fat, and carbohydrate metabolism and nervous system function; needed for oxygen use by cells	Meats, milk, poultry, eggs, whole-grain and enriched grain products, nuts
Vitamin B_6	Needed for protein metabolism; necessary for normal growth	Meats, fish, poultry, beans, grains, green leafy vegetables
Folate	Necessary for red blood cell development; needed for tissue growth and repair	Green leafy vegetables, oranges, beans, liver

(continued)

Table 5-1—*Continued*

Vitamin	Function	Food Sources
Vitamin B$_{12}$	Needed for new tissue growth, red blood cells, nervous system, and skin	Animal products—meat, fish, poultry, dairy foods
Biotin	Needed for normal metabolism of carbohydrates, fats, and protein	Widespread in foods
Pantothenate	Needed for normal metabolism of carbohydrates, fats, and protein	Widespread in foods—whole-grain and enriched grain products, vegetables, and meats
Vitamin C	Needed for building the material that holds cells together—collagen; necessary for healthy gums, teeth, and blood vessels	Citrus fruits, peppers, cabbage-family vegetables, strawberries, tomatoes
Vitamin D	Needed for calcium absorption; important for proper growth of bones and teeth	Body produces with sunlight, fortified milk, eggs, fish, liver
Vitamin E	Acts as antioxidant; protects cells from damage	Vegetable oils, green leafy vegetables, wheat germ, whole-grain products
Vitamin K	Aids in blood clotting	Cabbage-family vegetables, green leafy vegetables

- When cooking vegetables, steam or microwave them instead of boiling, to prevent vitamins from leaching into the cooking water.
- Store fruits and vegetables whole instead of in pieces.
- Keep fruit juices stored in airtight containers and freeze them whenever possible.

VITAMINS IN YOUR BODY

Vitamins get into your system in much the same way as carbohydrates or the other nutrients. Once your digestive tract absorbs the vitamins from a meal, along with the carbs, protein, fat, and minerals, it's time for these substances to get to work. For the most part, the water-soluble vitamins move quickly to all parts of your body, doing their job primarily in processing the other nutrients from the meal. Your body does not have the ability to store these vitamins for later use, so within 24 to 48 hours, the water-soluble vitamins are turned over—that is, they are broken down into useful elements or excreted from your body. Fast turnover explains why most people excrete brightly colored urine within 8 hours after taking a vitamin pill. The excess water-soluble vitamins spill into the urine, going unused.

Fat-soluble vitamins, on the other hand, aren't disposed of as quickly and can be stored for later use in various parts of the body, particularly the liver. In fact, your liver has about a one-to-two year supply of vitamin A. Because of this storage ability, you can go on for extended periods of time eating a vitamin A–poor diet without seeing the ill effects of fat-soluble vitamin deficiencies. However, water-soluble vitamin deficiency symptoms show up after about 40 to 60 days on a vitamin-deficient diet. This difference between fat-soluble and water-soluble vitamin storage explains why taking excessive amounts of vitamins A and D (fat-soluble) can lead to serious toxicity problems. They accumulate in your body with potentially harmful consequences. (More on this later).

In "RDA: What It Really Means" on page 161, I'll show you how much of each vitamin you require and explain the potential need for a vitamin supplement. But for now, remember that each vitamin has a unique role in your body, and that each one works *with* the food you eat to keep you healthy.

MEET THE MINERALS

Just like the vitamins, minerals keep your metabolism clicking along by assisting in chemical reactions. Minerals also keep you in balance by controlling your body's pH (acid level) and water balance. Unlike vitamins, however, minerals give your body shape by providing structure to bones and teeth. And unlike any other nutrient, minerals are inorganic—simple elements that originate from the earth's soil and water. Minerals are so simple in their nature that your body does not metabolize them—that is, it doesn't arrange and rearrange their chemical structure as it does other nutrients.

Frequently, minerals are grouped into two categories: *major* and *trace* minerals, based on how much of a particular mineral is present in your body and needed in the diet. For example, you have about 1,000 grams (two pounds) of calcium in your body and require about 1 gram daily. On the other hand, the total amount of the ten trace minerals in your body would fit neatly into a soupspoon. Your daily requirement for these trace minerals adds up to a tiny fraction of your calcium requirement.

No matter how much you may need of a particular mineral or what level of it is present in your body, each mineral plays a significant but different role in your health and performance. Zinc, for example, is a key player in fighting illness and in wound healing. On the other hand, calcium not only makes up much of the structure of bones and teeth, it is also vital for muscle action during exercise.

Check Tables 5-2 and 5-3 for more on specific mineral action in the body. At present, 15 minerals are known to be essential in the diet, but ongoing research suggests that other minerals like boron and nickel, still labeled "nonessential," may indeed have vital roles in health and performance.

MINERALS IN FOOD

Virtually all foods and beverages—even water—contain a mix of minerals. Since minerals originate from soil and water, foods like vegetables, fruits, and grains (or products made from animals that eat plants and drink water) are great sources of minerals. Eating a wide variety of foods ensures sufficient intake of the minerals, just as it does vitamins.

Some foods, however, are better sources than others for a particular mineral because it is more "available"—more of the mineral is able to enter the body or be absorbed—from the foods. About 30 percent of the iron in red meat can be absorbed, as opposed to less than 10 percent of the iron in grain foods such as bread.

Mineral levels in foods can drop much the same way vitamin content does. Since minerals dissolve well in water, soaking vegetables, immersing foods in water when you cook them, or draining the juices from foods results in minerals lost from food you finally eat. However, minerals are chemically very stable, so high-heat cooking methods like baking, steaming, barbecuing, or microwaving don't alter mineral levels in foods.

MINERALS IN THE BODY

Minerals make their way into your system along with the carbs, protein, and fat from a meal. But depending upon which mineral it is, only 5 to 60 percent of it actually becomes part of your body. Physical properties inherent in a particular food are largely to blame for this poor absorption rate. For example, fiber in whole grains, tannins in coffee and tea, and oxalate found in spinach and other vegetables all inhibit (but do not prevent) iron from entering your body.

Partially alleviating this problem is your body's own ability to increase the absorption of certain minerals when they are needed for normal functioning. For example, the intestines take up more calcium, zinc, and iron when your need for any one of these minerals increases. Then, suppose your blood level of iron was to fall, more iron would be taken up from the intestines in an effort to correct the deficiency.

Once minerals enter your bloodstream, they quickly move through the watery parts of your body and end up in every cell to perform vital tasks. You continually lose minerals from your body, primarily in urine and sweat. Since many of the minerals are "stored" in the body to cover these losses, you may not notice the consequences of mineral loss immediately. But diseases like iron-deficiency anemia and osteoporosis develop over many months or years when mineral stores become drained.

Table 5-2 *ELEMENTAL NEEDS: THE MAJOR MINERALS*

Mineral	Function	Food Sources
Calcium	Used for bone and tooth structure, muscle contraction, blood clotting, and healthy nerve function	Milk and milk products, green leafy vegetables, sardines with bones, tofu
Chloride	Works with sodium to maintain fluid balance; aids in digestion	Foods with salt (sodium chloride)
Magnesium	Aids in normal nerve and muscle function; is part of bone mineral structure	Green vegetables, beans, nuts, cocoa and chocolate, grains
Phosphorus	Combines with calcium for healthy bone and tooth structure; used in energy metabolism; is part of every cell's genetic material	Meats, fish, poultry, milk, beans
Potassium	Works with sodium to maintain fluid balance; helps control acid balance in body	Whole foods— vegetables, fruits, meats, milk
Sodium	Vital for fluid balance and normal nervous system function	Salt, processed foods, soy sauce and other seasonings

Table 5-3 *ELEMENTAL NEEDS: TRACE MINERALS*

Mineral	Function	Food Sources
Chromium	Needed for carbohydrate metabolism	Whole grains, vegetables, organ meats, brewer's yeast
Copper	Essential for blood cell and connective tissue formation	Grains, shellfish, organ meats, legumes
Fluoride	Makes tooth enamel more resistant to decay	Water containing flourides, fish, tea
Iodine	Part of thyroid hormone controlling basal metabolism and weight gain	Milk, grains, iodized salt
Iron	Important for oxygen transport and energy metabolism	Red meat, poultry, fish, green leafy vegetables, whole grains, legumes
Manganese	Used in bone and connective tissue formation, carbohydrate and fat metabolism	Spinach, pumpkin, nuts, legumes, tea
Molybdenum	Needed for nitrogen metabolism	Unprocessed grains and vegetables
Selenium	With vitamin E, helps protect body tissue from oxidation and other aging processes	Grains, meat, fish, poultry
Zinc	Used for wound healing, growth, appetite, sperm production	Seafood, meats, nuts, legumes

RDA: WHAT IT REALLY MEANS

You know vitamins and minerals are vital for top-notch performance and good health, but how much of each do you need to be at your best? While you may be aware that the RDAs (Recommended Dietary Allowances) for vitamins and minerals exist, what do these numbers actually mean to you?

For example, when is the RDA enough for your vitamin and mineral needs, and what happens to you and your performance when you don't routinely meet your requirement? The answers to these questions, plus how best to get needed vitamins and minerals with the Top Ten Super Foods for vitamin/mineral nutrition, are next.

THE ABCs OF THE RDAs

Historically, the RDAs have been around since 1943, when they were established to ensure adequate nutrition for the U.S. soldiers fighting in World War II. They have been updated nine times since to reflect new information on nutrient needs. Now the RDAs are used by the public as a nutritional "rule of thumb" for required vitamins and minerals as well as for proteins and calories (energy). The National Research Council's extensive information on vitamin and mineral needs is the basis for recommended intake that covers nearly all healthy people in the population.

Crucial to understanding what the RDAs mean is the fact that the numbers do not represent minimum, or even average, requirements for nutrients. Instead, the RDA for a particular nutrient reflects the average need plus an additional amount to cover the varying individual needs among the population. Also, the RDAs take into account the vitamin and mineral losses from foods that occur during processing and cooking. And for certain minerals like iron, the RDA value reflects the body's relative lack of ability to absorb them from foods ingested.

In addition to these considerations, the RDAs are also based on age, gender, and body size, since these factors influence vitamin and mineral needs. Specific RDAs are set for pregnant and nursing women. In all, there are 17 categories of RDAs based on age and gender. However, many health professionals criticize the current RDAs (1989) for not dividing the over-51-year-old category into two: 51 to 69 years and 70-plus. New evidence suggests that the nutritional needs of a 51-year-old may be different from those of an 80-year-old. Perhaps future revisions will reflect these findings.

Taking all the safety factors, age, and gender adjustments into consideration, you could say that if the RDAs err, they err on the side of generosity. In fact, if you average less than the RDA for a particular vitamin or mineral (about 70 to 75 percent) there is no cause for concern, because your actual needs are most likely being met anyway. It's also important to point out that the RDAs should not be looked at as daily requirements you must meet, but rather levels you average over several days. In fact, on some days you may take in less than half the suggested amounts, while on other days you may go well beyond what is recommended.

If you're beginning to think it takes a college degree in nutrition and a specialized food composition book to know how much of a particular vitamin or mineral you get from a food—relax. Meeting your RDA for many of the nutrients is actually quite easy. Table 5-4 suggests how much of a particular food provides a significant amount of the RDA (10 percent or more) of a specific vitamin or mineral.

WHEN THE RDAs ARE NOT ENOUGH

There are situations, however, when the vitamin and mineral RDAs do not cover your needs. A basic assumption in the establishment of the RDAs is that an individual is healthy: No serious illness or injuries are present that would change nutrient needs. For example, since zinc is vital to wound healing, someone badly injured—suffering from burns or serious scrapes—would need additional zinc for optimal recovery. How *much* extra would depend upon the seriousness of the injury. Hospitalized individuals are typically given supplemental vitamins and minerals to cover increased needs.

The most recent edition of the RDAs has established a separate recommended intake of vitamin C for smokers. Enough evidence exists to show that smokers metabolize vitamin C more quickly

(continued on page 166)

Table 5-4 *HOW MUCH IS ENOUGH?*

Here are the Recommended Dietary Allowances (RDA) for vitamins and minerals, along with foods that supply at least 10 percent of your requirement.

Nutrient	RDA		Foods Providing at Least 10% of RDA
	Men	Women	
Vitamins			
Vitamin A	1,000 retinol equivalents (R.E.)	800 retinol equivalents (R.E.)	½ carrot, 1 cup milk, ½ mango, ½ cup cooked bok choy
Thiamin (B_1)	1.5 mg	1.0 mg	¼ cup wheat germ, 3 oz. roasted ham, 1 cup oatmeal, 1 cup cooked peas
Riboflavin (B_2)	1.7 mg	1.3 mg	1 cup milk, 1 cup cooked beet greens, 1 cup raw mushrooms
Niacin (B_3)	19 mg	15 mg	3 oz. cooked beef or poultry, 3 oz. broiled fish, 1 baked potato
Vitamin B_6	2 mg	1.6 mg	1 banana, 3 oz. canned tuna, 1 cup watermelon, 10 dried figs
Folate	200 mcg	180 mcg	1 cup cooked broccoli, 1 cup bean sprouts, ½ cantaloupe, 1 cup pinto beans

(continued)

POWER FOODS: THE FACTS

Table 5-4—Continued

Nutrient	RDA		Foods Providing at Least 10% of RDA
	Men	Women	
Vitamins			
Vitamin B$_{12}$	2 mcg	2 mcg	3 oz. cooked meat, 1 cup milk, 1 egg
Vitamin C	60 mg	60 mg	1 tomato, ½ green pepper, ¼ cantaloupe, ½ orange
Vitamin D	5 mcg	5 mcg	3 oz. broiled salmon, 1 egg, 1 cup fortified milk
Vitamin E	10 mg	8 mg	¼ cup wheat germ, 1 Tbsp. corn oil or safflower oil, 1 Tbsp. ranch-style salad dressing
Vitamin K	80 mcg	65 mcg	1 cup cooked collard greens, 1 cup raw cabbage
Minerals			
Calcium	800 mg	800 mg	1 cup cooked broccoli, 1 cup milk (30%), 1 oz. Swiss cheese, 3 oz. canned salmon
Chloride	750 mg*	750 mg*	1 tsp. salt, soy sauce
Chromium	50–200 mg†	50–200 mg†	3 oz. cooked lean beef or poultry
Copper	1.5–3.0 mg†	1.5–3.0 mg†	3 oz. cooked lean beef or poultry
Fluoride	1.5–4.0 mg†	1.5–4.0 mg†	1 cup tea or fluoridated water, 3 oz. broiled seafood
Iodine	150 mcg	150 mcg	½ tsp. iodized salt, 3 oz. broiled seafood
Iron	10 mg	15 mg	1 cup cooked kidney beans, 1 baked potato,

Mineral			Good Food Sources
Magnesium	350 mg	280 mg	1 cup prune juice, 3 oz. lean beef
Manganese	2.0–5.0 mg†	2.0–5.0 mg†	1 cup cooked beet greens, 3 oz. tofu, ¼ cup wheat germ, 1 cup cooked kidney beans
Molybdenum	75–250 mcg†	75–250 mcg†	1 cup cooked spinach, 1 cup cooked beans, 1 cup cooked pumpkin
Phosphorus	800 mg	800 mg	1 cup cooked whole grains, 1 cup cooked broccoli; 1 cup milk, 3 oz. roasted turkey, ½ cup tofu, 3 oz. broiled lean beef
Potassium	2,000 mg*	2,000 mg*	1 banana, 1 cup winter squash, 1 tomato, 1 baked potato
Selenium	70 mcg	55 mcg	3 oz. broiled seafood, 3 oz. cooked lean beef, 1 cup cooked whole grains
Sodium	500 mg*	500 mg*	3 oz. water-packed tuna, 1 cup salted popcorn, 1 cup ready-to-eat cereal (many processed foods exceed minimum requirement)
Zinc	15 mg	12 mg	¼ cup wheat germ, 3 oz. roasted turkey, 3 oz. lean beef, 1 cup black-eyed peas

SOURCES: National Academy of Sciences, *Recommended Dietary Allowances* (Washington, D.C.: National Academy Press, 1989).

Composition of Foods, Agriculture Handbook No. 8 (Washington, D.C.: U.S. Government Printing Office, 1975).

*Estimated minimum requirement, *Food and Nutrition Board,* 1989.

†Estimated safe and adequate daily intakes, *Food and Nutrition Board,* 1989.

than nonsmokers do and are more likely to deplete blood and tissue levels of vitamin C. Beyond smoking, other considerations, such as the use of medicines that change vitamin or mineral needs, are not taken into account in the RDAs. Contact your physician if you are concerned that any medications you are taking negatively impact on your vitamin or mineral needs.

WHAT THE RDAs MEAN TO ATHLETES

While the current RDAs are adjusted for age and gender, they make no provisions for special demands of exercise. People are presumed to have "typical" activity levels, but the consequence

---

Table 5-5 *EVERYDAY MEDICATIONS THAT INTERFERE WITH VITAMINS AND MINERALS*

Medicine	Effect
Antacids	Increase loss of phosphorus and destruction of thiamin
Antibiotics	(Depends upon type of antibiotic.) Decrease absorption of vitamins A and B_{12}, folate, iron, calcium, and zinc
Aspirin	Increases loss of vitamin C, thiamin, calcium, and iron
Diuretics (blood pressure control)	Increase loss of potassium, magnesium, calcium, and sodium
Laxatives (mineral oil)	Reduce the absorption of vitamins A, D, E, and K and calcium
Oral contraceptives	Alter use of riboflavin and B_6 and decrease absorption of folate

SOURCE: Adapted from F. J. Zeman, *Clinical Nutrition and Dietetics* (Lexington, Mass.: Collamore Educational Publishing, 1983).

---

of heavy exercise on vitamin and mineral needs is not considered. Therefore, some athletes feel justified in saying that the RDAs don't apply to them and that new recommended intakes should be determined for active people.

Exercise may affect the utilization, metabolism, or loss of vitamins and minerals. Sodium, for example, is lost in sweat at a rate of about 1 gram for every quart of sweat (0.5 gram is the minimum daily requirement). People who train for extended periods of time, or who sweat heavily, run the risk of dangerously depleting body sodium levels, which could be life-threatening.

Iron and riboflavin needs may also rise with heavy training. During a workout or competition, your body relies on B vitamins, such as riboflavin, and iron to help liberate energy from food to power your working muscles. Research shows that the RDA for riboflavin of 0.6 milligrams per 1,000 calories in the diet may be insufficient when training. While supplemental riboflavin doesn't appear to boost performance, 1.1 milligrams per 1,000 calories in the diet is suggested to meet the demands of exercise.

Regular exercisers, particularly women and endurance athletes, run the risk of iron deficiency. Iron is responsible for releasing energy from food as well as for carrying oxygen to working muscles. Increased iron losses due to exercise or insufficient iron in the diet may be responsible for performance problems seen in some athletes with poor iron status. (See "Pumping Iron" later in this chapter.)

On the other hand, scientists do not agree that exercise markedly affects the needs for iron, riboflavin, or any other vitamin or mineral. Since the RDAs have built-in margins of safety, many researchers claim any increased need due to exercise is probably covered if you consume at, or near, the level of the RDA.

I recommend that people who exercise regularly, or who train and race frequently, consume 100 percent of the RDA for every vitamin and mineral. Since active people generally eat more food than others, this should not be difficult. Yet it's difficult to know what your specific vitamin or mineral intake is. A computerized diet analysis performed by a qualified dietitian/nutritionist, however, can help you determine your approximate intake of most vitamins and minerals.

But rather than center your diet around the RDAs, use a simpler approach: Eat a diet rich in nutrient-dense foods. In short, my Power Diet, loaded with a plentiful supply of fruits and vegetables, grains, and low-fat protein foods (lean meats, low-fat dairy products, and vegetable protein sources) will supply you with the vitamin and mineral nutrition you need to stay in top form. "Power Menu Plan" on page 172 shows one day's power menu containing 100 percent RDA or more of most vitamins and minerals.

HOW DO YOU KNOW YOU'RE GETTING ENOUGH NUTRIENTS?

If you're like most people, you have some concern about whether you're getting enough vitamins and minerals in your diet. Perhaps you have an erratic eating schedule, or you fear that processed foods are robbing you of precious nutrients. Even if you average an intake of 100 percent, or even more, of the RDA for vitamins and minerals, it is still unsettling to realize that your body might not have the nourishment it needs for top performance.

Signs of vitamin and mineral deficiencies serve as warnings that you are short of these precious nutrients. Table 5-6 lists symptoms typically seen in people who don't meet their personal requirements. As you can see, the consequences of deficiency can be devastating, but fortunately, problems brought on by severe nutrient deficiencies are rare.

In general, these deficiency problems occur when vitamin and mineral intakes routinely fall 20 to 30 percent below the RDA. People who eat a well-balanced diet, even going for frequent periods without wholesome foods, rarely suffer from vitamin and mineral deficiencies. It is alcoholics, chronically malnourished individuals, those on various medications that change vitamin and mineral needs, or others with altered nutrient requirements who run the risk of deficiency problems.

But what are the consequences of routinely falling short of meeting vitamin and mineral needs? Will your performance on the job and in the gym be affected by a marginal intake of vitamins and minerals? This is an area of debate in vitamin-and-mineral nutrition. Some scientists argue that unless you show

Table 5-6 *THE SIGNS OF TOO LITTLE*

Nutrient	Deficiency Symptoms
Vitamins	
Vitamin A	Night blindness, anemia, depressed immune system, respiratory infections, hair follicles become plugged with keratin (hard and white), total blindness
Thiamin (B_1)	Weakness, fatigue, painful muscles progressing to paralysis and heart failure
Riboflavin (B_2)	Skin rash, bright red tongue, cracks at corners of mouth
Niacin (B_3)	Diarrhea, severe cracking and darkening of skin, weakness and delirium
Vitamin B_6	Anemia, skin rash, muscle spasms and convulsions
Folate	Anemia, diarrhea, fatigue and depression, smooth, bright red tongue
Vitamin B_{12}	Anemia, fatigue, nerve degeneration that progresses to paralysis
Biotin and pantothenate	Deficiencies are extremely rare
Vitamin C	Bleeding gums, pinpoint hemorrhages under skin surface, weakness, joint pain, impaired wound healing, depression, scurvy
Vitamin D	Retarded bone growth and stunting in children, poor formation of teeth, soft bone fractures in adults, muscle spasms
Vitamin E	Anemia from weak red blood cells, weakness and muscle pain
Vitamin K	Inability to clot blood
Minerals	
Calcium	Poor bone growth in children and weak, brittle bones in adults (osteoporosis)
Copper	Anemia, growth problems in children

(continued)

Table 5-6—*Continued*

Nutrient	Deficiency Symptoms
Minerals	
Fluoride	Increased susceptibility to tooth decay, possibly associated with development of osteoporosis
Iodine	Enlarged thyroid gland, sluggishness and weight gain, mental retardation and stunted growth in newborns of deficient mothers
Iron	Anemia, fatigue, decreased physical performance
Magnesium	Feelings of weakness, muscle tremors, convulsions
Potassium	Muscle weakness, fatigue, paralysis
Selenium	Heart disease called Keshan disease (tissue breakdown)
Zinc	Delay in sexual development, poor wound healing, depressed immune response

NOTE: These deficiency signs are not meant to be used as a diagnostic tool. Please consult your physician with questions regarding possible vitamin and mineral deficiencies.

the classic symptoms of vitamin or mineral deficiency, you are adequately nourished. But others argue that simply feeling under the weather may be a sign of marginal vitamin or mineral deficiency.

Accumulating evidence suggests that marginal vitamin and mineral status may indeed be to blame for increased susceptibility to disease and infection, slowed recovery from injuries or illness, and even problems with thinking ability, fatigue, and physical stamina.

Assessment of marginal vitamin and mineral status can be made through blood tests and other laboratory measurements. But don't rely on "health clinics" that perform questionable tests (hair analysis, for example) to evaluate your supply. Check with your physician to get an accurate picture of your vitamin and mineral levels.

STANDOUT VITAMINS AND MINERALS

It is necessary to consume every one of the essential vitamins and minerals for good health and top-notch performance. However, certain vitamins and minerals stand out as having health benefits beyond their particular biochemical function in the body. Lower risks for chronic diseases like cancer, heart disease, and osteoporosis have been linked to diets rich in specific vitamins and minerals. For example, studies show that people with a regular intake of foods rich in vitamin C and beta-carotene (the fruit and vegetable form of vitamin A) have a lower incidence of certain types of cancer.

As we age, we fall victim to the ravages of modern life, such as air pollution and other environmental contaminants; even time itself impacts on our health. These standout vitamins and minerals may protect us from some of the killer diseases that are linked to our lifestyles and may even improve the quality of our life through better health.

These health-promoting nutrients are listed below with information on how they work to protect your body. While there's no agreement in the scientific community as to how much of each vitamin and mineral you need for all these benefits, your diet is the best source of supply. Most research links foods rich in these nutrients with some health benefit.

Vitamin C. Vitamin C acts as an antioxidant, protecting your body from substances and chemical reactions that damage tissues. High intake of vitamin C is linked to a decreased risk of certain types of cancer as well as decreased incidence of cataract formation (the leading cause of blindness in people over age 65).

Best food sources: Citrus fruits, green and other peppers, broccoli, tomatoes, strawberries, potatoes.

Vitamin A/beta-carotene. Vitamin A helps prevent the formation of free radicals, substances that damage cell membranes and promote formation and growth of cancer. Beta-carotene, a pigment that gives many fruits and vegetables their yellow-to-red color, is converted to vitamin A inside the body. Diets rich in beta-carotene and vitamin A have been shown to lower cancer risk.

Best food sources: Yellow-orange fruits and green and yellow-

POWER MENU PLAN

Here's a day's worth of meals and snacks that supply the vitamins and minerals you need for stamina and performance.

Breakfast

> Bagel with 1 tablespoon jam and 1 teaspoon margarine
>
> 1 cup whole-grain cereal (NutriGrain) with 1 cup low-fat (2 percent) milk
>
> 6 ounces orange juice

Lunch

> Tuna sandwiches: 4 slices whole-grain bread and 3 ounces water-packed tuna mixed with 2 teaspoons mayonnaise
>
> 1 carrot
>
> 1 cup mixed fruit: strawberries, kiwifruit, and nectarines
>
> 12 ounces iced tea
>
> 4 fig bars

Snack

> 2 ounces pretzels
>
> 1 apple

Dinner

> 1 cup steamed broccoli
>
> 2 cups mixed salad with 1 tablespoon oil and vinegar dressing
>
> 1 cup cooked pasta with 1⅔ cup red sauce with oysters (3 ounces cooked)
>
> 1 cup skim milk
>
> 1 slice peach pie

Snack

> 2 cups air-popped popcorn
>
> 12 ounces fruit-flavored mineral water

Analysis

Total calories:2,900. Distribution: 65 percent carbohydrate, 15 percent protein, 20 percent fat. Supplies 100 percent of the RDA for vitamins A, B_6, B_{12}, C, and E, thiamin, riboflavin, niacin, folate, calcium, iron, and zinc.

orange vegetables such as apricots, peaches, cantaloupes, carrots, winter squashes, broccoli, spinach, collard greens, beet greens.

Vitamin E. Another antioxidant, vitamin E specifically positions itself on the surface of cell membranes to fight free-radical attacks that could damage cells. Increased exposure to air pollution and other environmental contaminants may call for additional vitamin E to combat the damaging effect of these substances. Also, some studies show that vitamin E status may be diminished with exercise, particularly at high altitude. Age-related changes such as cataract formation have also been linked to low vitamin E intake.

Best food sources: Vegetable oils, salad dressings made with vegetable oils, whole grains, wheat germ, leafy green vegetables such as spinach.

Selenium. Selenium works with vitamin E in protecting cell membranes from free-radical attack. Inadequate intake of this mineral is linked to an increased risk of cancer. However, selenium supplements are not recommended because as little as two to three times the RDA can be toxic.

Best food sources: Meats and seafood as well as grains and vegetables (however, selenium content of foods depends upon selenium content of soil and/or water where they are harvested).

Calcium. Calcium is well known as the mineral crucial for healthy bone. Sufficient calcium intake throughout life is the best protection against the debilitating bone disease osteoporosis, common in women over the age of 55. After about age 35, your bones start to lose calcium, and they can become weak and susceptible to fractures. Adequate calcium intake before age 35 is critical for achieving optimal bone size and, from then on, for maintaining bone mass. A good supply of calcium is also linked to a reduced risk for high blood pressure, one of the leading factors in heart disease. Bear in mind that good levels of vitamin D help in calcium absorption.

Best food sources: Low-fat and nonfat dairy products (milk, yogurt, frozen yogurt, ice milk, cheese), tofu, green leafy vegetables (bok choy, turnip greens), salmon with bones, blackstrap molasses.

TOP TEN SUPER FOODS

Get what you need in the way of the standout vitamins and minerals—vitamins A, C, and E, plus selenium and calcium—and other key nutrients with my Top Ten Super Foods. Before you consider a supplement, check out the number of foods that pack a wealth of vitamin and mineral nutrition. Many of these Super Foods supply more than the RDA for certain vitamins and minerals.

The old adage still holds: Eat a variety of foods to get all the nutrients you need. But for super nutrition, include these blockbuster foods on a regular basis.

Broccoli. This wonder vegetable supplies these nutritional RDA needs: 120 percent of vitamin C, 35 percent of vitamin A (as beta-carotene), 10 percent of vitamin E, 10 percent of calcium, 50 percent of folate, and 10 percent of iron, per cup cooked. In addition, broccoli is from the cruciferous vegetable family, the frequent consumption of which is linked to a reduced cancer risk.

Eat broccoli raw or steamed; use as a vegetable side dish, raw for dipping, in stir-fries, or in soups and casseroles.

Green pepper. This versatile veggie is packed with vitamin C—over 200 percent of the RDA in one raw pepper. Peppers also supply just under 10 percent of the RDA for vitamin A (as beta-carotene) and iron. Other peppers—yellow, red, or hot varieties—are also great sources of these nutrients.

Peppers are tasty raw or in stir-fries; use raw for dipping, or try a variety of types in soups, stews, and sauces.

Nonfat yogurt. If you're looking for a fat-free calcium source, this is it. One cup of nonfat yogurt contains 30 percent of the calcium RDA, along with 30 percent of the riboflavin and 50 percent of the vitamin B_{12} RDA.

Blend yogurt with fruit for a quick-to-make drink; mix with herbs for a vegetable dip; or stir into soups for a nutritious "cream" soup.

Wheat germ. The portion of the wheat kernel that was meant to sprout into a wheat plant is loaded with goodies: One-quarter cup provides 40 percent of the selenium RDA, 30 percent of the zinc RDA, 50 percent of the folate RDA, 17 percent of iron needs, and over 100 percent of the suggested manganese requirement.

Use wheat germ to top off your morning cereal; mix into bread dough, muffins, and cake batters; stir into casseroles; and add to blended drinks for a nutty flavor.

Swiss chard. This unpretentious leafy vegetable is packed with many of the standout vitamins and minerals: One cup cooked has over 50 percent of the vitamin A requirement (as beta-carotene), 50 percent of the vitamin C RDA, and 10 percent of vitamin E and calcium needs. Chard also supplies 40 percent of the magnesium RDA and 25 percent of the iron requirement, along with about half of the suggested potassium intake.

Chard does well in soups, stews, and casseroles, or use raw in salads mixed with other greens.

Extralean beef. While you think of beef as a protein source, a three-ounce cooked serving supplies over 100 percent of the RDA for vitamin B_{12}, 28 percent of the RDA for vitamin B_6, 37 percent of the RDA for selenium, 19 percent of iron needs, and 37 percent of the zinc RDA.

Use beef in stir-fries (use a nonstick pan), or broil, bake, or microwave instead of frying.

Kidney beans. Besides being a great source of fiber, beans are also loaded with minerals: A one-cup serving of cooked kidney beans supplies 23 percent of the magnesium RDA, 35 percent of the iron requirement, 12 percent of the zinc RDA, 25 percent of the suggested copper intake, along with 100 percent of the folate RDA.

Use beans as a side dish, combine them with a grain for a complete protein, or add them to soups, stews, and casseroles.

Cantaloupe. This fruit is a wealth of nutrients, supplying 50 percent of the vitamin A (as beta-carotene) and over 100 percent of the vitamin C requirements in a one-cup serving. That's not all; this same serving has about 50 percent of the potassium needs and 10 percent of the folate requirement.

Use cantaloupe on its own or in a fruit salad; blend it with other fruit for a power smoothie.

Oysters. A three-ounce serving of canned oysters supplies an unbelievable 400 percent of the zinc RDA, 800 percent of the vitamin B_{12} RDA, 40 percent of the iron requirement, 13 percent of the magnesium RDA, and over 100 percent of the suggested copper intake.

Add oysters to ready-made spaghetti sauce, soups, stews, and casseroles; or blend them with low-fat cottage cheese, yogurt, and herbs for a tasty power dip. Note, however, that it's not wise to eat oysters raw: Cook them to remove potential bacterial or parasitic problems.

Potato. This popular vegetable has a lot to offer: One baked potato with the skin provides 50 percent of the vitamin C requirement, 18 percent of the iron RDA, about 50 percent of potassium needs, 18 percent of the niacin RDA, and 30 percent of the suggested copper intake.

This vegetable can do almost anything: Use it as a main dish topped with steamed vegetables and low-fat cheese; use as a side dish steamed or microwaved; add to soups and stews; mash cooked potatoes and use in muffins, breads, and rolls.

WHY AM I SO TIRED?

You've been there before—you've had an unrelenting day at work or in a marathon-like workout, and you feel fatigued, dog tired. You know that a good night's sleep or a bit of relaxation usually restores your energy level. But sometimes the fatigue lingers—maybe a week, a month, or even longer. You can't help but wonder what's making you feel so weak and tired. And you worry.

Before you self-diagnose and consider taking any action, I encourage you to see your physician if you're suffering from chronic fatigue. It's particularly important to do so if your fatigue is accompanied by a sore throat, aching muscles, swollen lymph nodes, and headaches.

WHAT CAUSES FATIGUE?

You certainly know it when you have it, but fatigue shows no visible marks and it's hard to know how serious it is. As for its causes—there are many. Temporary fatigue, for example, can be brought on by any hard physical effort or by mental strain. Chronic fatigue, however, has more elusive beginnings that frustrate both the investigating physician and his patient. While there is a chronic fatigue syndrome identified as a medical condition that has been linked to a specific virus, most individuals who suffer from general fatigue go on with their lives, performing in slow motion. There are, however, links between vitamin and mineral deficiencies (and overdoses) and chronic fatigue.

Vitamin deficiency symptoms, for example, don't emerge overnight. It takes a period of months, during which time feelings of fatigue and weakness are common. As some tissue in your body becomes depleted of a vitamin, various biochemical changes take place that can cause you to sense a general lack of well-being before any specific vitamin deficiency signs are seen. In cases of mild thiamin deficiency, for example, individuals have no physically apparent signs of deficiency, such as nerve damage, but they do complain about feelings of lethargy, fatigue, and a loss of appetite.

Mineral deficiencies can also result in chronic fatigue. A classic example is iron deficiency, which saps the blood's ability to carry oxygen to tissues, leaving you exhausted at the slightest exertion. Many people suffer from iron-poor blood and, as a consequence, operate at less than optimal levels, letting their work and exercise suffer. If chronic fatigue is plaguing you, it could be due to iron deficiency. But before you consider iron dosing, read the next section, "Pumping Iron," so you can do what's best for you.

Fatigue is also linked to vitamin and mineral overdosing. One sign of taking too much vitamin C, for example, is a feeling of fatigue sometimes accompanied by nausea. Magnesium overdose can also cause extreme fatigue. High levels of magnesium typically aren't possible through diet, but certain antacids may supply more than the RDA in one dose. If you're a heavy user of antacids, check with your physician about potential problems.

PUMPING IRON

If you've ever felt dragged out and worn thin for more than a few days, you've probably considered taking an iron supplement to boost energy levels. You're not alone. Many athletes, as well as ordinary people on the job, have turned to iron dosing as a way to beat chronic fatigue. But should you take iron as a precautionary measure to stay ahead of your exhausting schedule?

No. For most people—athlete or not—taking extra iron is not only unnecessary but unwise. Iron supplements can cause intestinal discomfort and alter nutrient use by the body. Also, research indicates that iron supplements may be linked to cancer.

However, iron supplements do have their place. Endurance athletes who suffer from iron deficiency need to take extra iron to recover lost levels of performance. The decision to use iron supplements in such cases should be based on sound information and complete medical testing.

IRON BASICS

Proper levels of iron must be maintained for consistent training and successful performance. Found in the hemoglobin in healthy red blood cells, this essential mineral delivers oxygen to exercising muscles. Iron also plays a key role in energy metabolism of working muscle tissues. If your iron status is depressed, you may develop anemia—a condition identified by low blood hemoglobin levels. Marked by sluggishness and fatigue, anemia causes the blood to lose some of its ability to carry oxygen to working muscles.

Anemia brought on by iron depletion occurs more frequently in runners than in the general population. Reasons range from blood loss in the urine to increased breakdown of red blood cells due to foot pounding, as well as the obvious—poor dietary intake.

A few years ago, researchers were astonished by the large number of seemingly anemic athletes. But now we know that low hemoglobin values (less than 13 grams per deciliter for men, less than 12 for women) don't necessarily indicate anemia, especially for athletes. Hard training triggers a unique physiological response that can cloud the hemoglobin picture. To meet the demands of exercise, athletes develop greater blood volume. This adaptation effectively dilutes the percentage of red blood cells, which results in lower hemoglobin readings. If interpreted incorrectly, low hemoglobin in an athlete may be considered anemia when, in fact, it may indicate increased blood volume and a high level of fitness.

So if your hemoglobin shows up low, you should probably ask for additional tests to further evaluate your iron status and risk for anemia. Measuring ferritin, the body's primary iron-storage protein, will indicate if iron stores are sapped even when hemoglobin levels are normal. Transferrin, another iron indicator that transports iron in the blood, can also be studied in a routine blood test.

If you suffer from chronic fatigue, weakness, and irritability—key symptoms of iron-deficiency anemia—don't hesitate to make an appointment for a blood workup. Armed with the results of a comprehensive blood test, you and your doctor can better decide if you need iron supplements.

IRON IRONY

While supplemental iron will boost sagging iron stores and alleviate anemia, you should not think of piling on iron as a preventive measure. Iron supplements contain anywhere from 30 to 200 milligrams, so far above the RDA of 10 milligrams for men and 15 milligrams for women that they might cause adverse side effects—most notably, constipation and diarrhea. The higher the dose, the worse the discomfort. Nausea and stomach pain can also occur, but they last only until iron use is discontinued.

Furthermore, excessive iron intake inhibits the absorption of zinc. Because the body absorbs both iron and zinc through the intestinal tract, excess iron takes precedence, virtually bumping zinc out of the way. More than 25 milligrams of iron at one meal is sufficient to cause problems with zinc absorption. Also, since research has shown that the zinc supply may be marginal for many athletes, iron supplements could be doing more harm than good.

Perhaps the most alarming news comes from researchers who link high iron stores to a greater risk of developing cancer. In a 10-year study, scientists looked at a large group of men and women who were initially cancer-free. The male subjects who developed cancer showed higher iron stores than the men who remained cancer-free. Cancer risk was 40 percent greater in men with high levels of iron. The link between cancer risk and high iron stores was weaker among female subjects, perhaps because women typically have lower iron stores and more rapid iron turnover than men. While this study established no definite link between iron in the diet and cancer risk, more research will follow to determine if excess dietary iron will be added to the long list of substances that may cause cancer.

Therefore, don't take extra iron unless you need to. Pregnant women and those who are diagnosed as iron-deficient will certainly benefit from extra iron, but for all others, a balanced diet should meet your daily needs. If you feel the need for "insurance," take a multivitamin/mineral supplement, which typically contains the 100 percent of your iron requirement. This is a safe amount for those who usually don't meet their iron needs through diet.

IRON BOOSTERS

The right foods will help you meet iron needs easily. The best form of dietary iron is *heme* iron, found in red meats, poultry (particularly dark meat), and fish. This iron is better utilized by your body than nonheme iron, found in fruits, vegetables, and whole grains. Nonheme iron is also found in animal products, particularly eggs and dairy foods.

Nonheme iron is plentiful in our diet but isn't absorbed well by the body; 5 to 10 percent of the nonheme iron is absorbed compared with 25 to 30 percent for heme iron. Furthermore, other dietary components may decrease nonheme iron absorption. Phytates, found in many vegetables and whole grains, can decrease iron absorption efficiency. Teas, coffees, and red wine contain tannins, which also bind iron and decrease its absorption by 40 to 80 percent.

Certain foods, however, can enhance the amount of iron absorbed from a meal. Vitamin C helps out significantly; having a glass of orange juice or a bowl of strawberries with your morning cereal can boost your iron utilization. Also, eating meats, fish, and poultry, even in small amounts, can boost the nonheme absorption of a meal. Check Table 5-7 for iron-rich foods to include daily.

THE BOTTOM LINE ON VITAMIN AND MINERAL SUPPLEMENTS

We've come all this way together, and you have a simple question left for me: "Do I need to take a vitamin and mineral supplement . . . just in case?" Many Americans already have made

Table 5-7 *IRON IN FOODS*

Food	Portion	Iron (mg)
Heme Iron Sources		
Liver, cooked	3 oz.	7
Canned oysters, cooked	3 oz.	6
Lean beef, cooked	3 oz.	3
Pork, cooked	3 oz.	2
Tuna, canned	3 oz.	2
Turkey, dark-meat, cooked	3 oz.	2
Chicken, dark-meat, cooked	3 oz.	1.5
Chicken, white-meat, cooked	3 oz.	1
Nonheme Iron Sources		
Ready-to-eat fortified breakfast cereal (e.g. Total, Kellogg's Raisin Bran)	¾ cup	18
Dried figs	10	4
Lentils, cooked	½ cup	3
Blackstrap molasses	1 Tbsp.	2
Kidney beans, cooked	½ cup	2
Spinach, cooked	½ cup	2
Wheat germ	¼ cup	2
Bread (enriched or whole-wheat)	1 slice	1
Enriched pasta, cooked	½ cup	1

SOURCE: Adapted from J. A. T. Pennington, *Bowes and Church's Food Values of Portions Commonly Used,* 15th ed. (Philadelphia: J. B. Lippincott, 1989).

the choice to use supplements; about five in ten adults take a vitamin and/or mineral supplement of some kind. I do, and I will show you why I made that decision and how I use a supplement safely. I will also help you to decide whether a supplement is necessary for you.

DO *YOU* NEED TO TAKE A SUPPLEMENT?

I find that people take supplements for various reasons:
□ To make up for irregular eating habits—skipped meals, fre-

quent snacks, and poor meal planning
- [ ] As insurance against common illness—colds and flu
- [ ] To make up for presumed nutritional deficits in processed foods
- [ ] To help combat stress at work and home
- [ ] As prevention against long-term diseases like osteoporosis, cancer, and heart disease

None of these is a legitimate reason for vitamin/mineral supplementation. However, there are good reasons to take a supplement. But before you read on, keep in mind that no supplement can give your body 100 percent of what it needs to stay healthy. There are still other micronutrients science is studying right now to see if we need them and how much we might need. Obtaining vitamins and minerals from a variety of foods is unarguably the best and safest way to get what your body needs for top performance.

Missing a meal, for instance, will not significantly alter your vitamin or mineral status. It takes months and even years for an average healthy person to become vitamin or mineral deficient. Instead of being concerned with isolated eating incidents, such as a missed meal or an "unbalanced" meal that you consider upsetting to your nutritional level, look at the big picture. What you "average" in nutrition intake over weeks, months, and years has a far greater impact on your health and performance. Vitamins and minerals work with the food—the better the food, the healthier you can be.

VALID SUPPLEMENT SITUATIONS

As I pointed out in the section about the RDAs, your needs most likely are covered if you consume 70 to 100 percent of the RDA for that vitamin or mineral. However, there are special situations in which nutrient needs are altered above the RDA and a supplement may be beneficial. In addition to this, you may have difficulty meeting your vitamin and mineral requirements due to an inadequate diet for reasons other than poor food choices.

Here are some situations where a supplement may be beneficial. But before you supplement, read on about supplement safety and what type of supplement is best. Also, it's best to contact your physician about any special concerns you have before taking a supplement.

Chronic dieting. People who routinely eat less than 1,200 to 1,500 calories daily tend to fall short on meeting vitamin and mineral nutrient needs, since they are taking in so little food. Supplement type: multivitamin with minerals.

Food allergies. People with allergic reactions to certain types of foods, like wheat, fruit, or milk protein, need to compensate for missed nutrient intake. Supplement type: multivitamin with minerals or specific supplement as indicated by physician.

Pregnancy. Expectant women have increased needs for many nutrients which, except for iron, can be met through a balanced diet. Supplement type: multivitamin with minerals or iron supplement (see your physician).

Lactose intolerance. Many people, particularly Asians, Afro-Americans, Hispanics, and Native Americans, are unable to digest lactose, the sugar in milk. Avoiding dairy products means missing out on valuable sources of calcium and riboflavin. Unless alternate calcium-rich sources such as fortified soy milk are included, a supplement may be in order. Supplement type: multivitamin and/or calcium supplement.

Old age. People over the age of 65 may have altered nutrient requirements that are not reflected in the RDAs, which consider everyone over the age of 51 as a single group. Elderly individuals tend to have poor vitamin and mineral intake because they eat less than they did when they were younger: They may have difficulty eating at all due to ill-fitting dentures or have trouble shopping for food because of ailments such as arthritis that decrease their mobility. Supplement type: multivitamin with minerals (consult physician, since supplement toxicity problems may be more pronounced in the elderly).

Medications. Common drugs—oral contraceptives, antibiotics, and analgesics, for example—interfere with vitamin and mineral utilization. Supplement type: as indicated by specific drug; see your physician.

Frequent alcohol use. Alcohol from beer, wine, and liquor interferes with vitamin and mineral metabolism. It also increases the loss of certain minerals in the urine, such as zinc. Supplement type: multivitamin with minerals.

Vegetarian diets. Excluding meats, milk, eggs, and other animal products in a vegetarian diet must be met with alternate foods to replace missing nutrients. Intake of vitamin B_{12}, and possibly vitamin D, iron, and zinc, may be suboptimal, particularly for children and pregnant women. Supplement type: multivitamin with minerals.

NOT-NECESSARILY-A-SUPPLEMENT SITUATION

Other situations exist where a vitamin and/or mineral supplement is of questionable value. Emotional stress at work or at home, for example, is often cited as a reason for taking a supplement. Yet no evidence exists that nutrient needs increase during these times. Instead, poor nutrition intake due to erratic eating as a result of the stress may jeopardize your ability to cope with stressful situations as well as compromise your health.

Listed below are a few situations where supplements are frequently used to ward off illness or disease. While evidence exists linking a specific nutrient to a disorder, realize that supplementation will not necessarily prevent, lessen, or cure these diseases.

Osteoporosis. This disease, characterized by bones made weak and fragile through calcium loss, results from many factors occurring over the lifespan of an individual. Present calcium intake is just one consideration. Exercise habits, levels of the female hormone estrogen, past calcium intake, and other dietary factors all play a role in the development of this disease. For example, a sedentary lifestyle is linked to osteoporosis, and regular exercise can improve calcium deposition into bones, even after osteoporosis has occurred.

Instead of looking at the big picture of lifestyle and eating habits, people have made calcium supplements a cure-all for osteoporosis. The evidence to support supplementation as a solitary means of slowing bone mineral loss is weak. While calcium supplements may be an easy and reasonable way to insure adequate intake, a calcium pill does not represent prevention or cure of this chronic and debilitating disease.

Heart disease. Perhaps no ailment is more a product of our lifestyle than heart disease. Many factors combine to put us at risk for suffering a heart attack. Exercise habits, family history, blood cholesterol, gender, cigarette smoking, and high blood pressure are just a few factors that influence a person's risk. Certain minerals—calcium and magnesium—have been linked to lowering blood pressure. This has been interpreted by some to mean a supplement may lower blood pressure and prevent heart disease. Unfortunately, no convincing evidence supports mineral supplementation as a means of lowering heart disease risk.

Cancer. As pointed out earlier, various vitamins and minerals have a protective effect against certain types of cancer. Despite this association, supplementation has not been shown to decrease cancer risk. Instead, a diet rich in vitamins and minerals appears to be the best way to go. Perhaps an additional "protection factor" is present in the food along with vitamin/mineral combinations, protecting the body against cancer. This may help explain fiber's role in cancer prevention.

PICKING A SUPPLEMENT

Take a look at any supplement aisle at a drugstore or supermarket and you're likely to get confused and overwhelmed, if not frustrated, by all the possibilities. Your biggest concern in selecting a supplement should be to avoid potential hazards from overdosing. Next, you want to avoid choosing a supplement that has nonessential nutrients that add to the price but do nothing for your health.

Here are six guidelines to help you select a safe and beneficial supplement. (Remember: Act on the advice of a physician before taking supplements.)

1. Select a supplement that contains a balance of 100 to 150 percent of the RDA for each vitamin and mineral. A good multivitamin with minerals should contain the 13 recognized vitamins, iron, zinc, selenium, and possibly copper. Calcium and magnesium should also be present at approximately 10 to 25 percent of the RDA.

2. Avoid supplements for which there is a multiple dosage. If the label reads, "Four tablets daily supply . . . ," then think twice about buying this supplement. Chances are you will be paying more per daily dose, and you may find taking more than one pill a day a nuisance.

(continued on page 188)

Table 5-8 *VITAMIN AND MINERAL DOSING HAZARDS*

Nutrient	Overdosing Hazards/Symptoms	Purported Benefits from Megadosing
Vitamins		
Vitamin A	Nausea, loss of appetite, dry cracked skin, loss of hair, joint pain, severe headache, liver damage, possible death	Cancer prevention, acne treatment, improved eyesight
Thiamin (B_1)	None currently known	Increased physical performance
Riboflavin (B_2)	Bright yellow urine	Increased physical performance
Niacin (B_3)	Flushing and itchy skin, irritability, tachycardia	Treatment for mental illness; improves learning disabilities; treatment for heart disease, lowers blood cholesterol
Vitamin B_6	Neurological damage	Treatment for mental illness, menstrual edema, and premenstrual syndrome
Folate	Can mask diagnosis of pernicious anemia (vitamin B_{12} deficiency)	Boosts energy levels
Vitamin B_{12}	Unclear	Improved physical performance; treatment of multiple sclerosis; slows aging

	Symptoms of excess	Claims
Vitamin C	Nausea, diarrhea, kidney stones, potential mutagen	Prevention and cure of colds; immunity from diseases; cancer and heart disease treatment
Vitamin D	Growth retardation, calcium deposition in soft tissue, kidney damage	Builds stronger bones
Vitamin E	Fatigue, nausea, cramps, increased blood-fat levels; interferes with vitamins A and K metabolism (toxicity signs are rare)	Prevents, slows, or ameliorates aging, infertility, balding, diabetes, cancer, arthritis; improves sexual performance
Minerals		
Calcium	Kidney stones in susceptible individuals; interferes with absorption of iron and magnesium	Prevention of osteoporosis, high blood pressure, and heart disease
Iron	Constipation and/or diarrhea, iron overload in susceptible individuals (e.g. alcoholics)	Combats fatigue, prevents anemia
Magnesium	Lethargy, nausea, vomiting, kidney failure	Prevention of high blood pressure and heart disease
Selenium	Streaked fingernails, vomiting, nervous system disorders	Cancer prevention
Zinc	Nausea, diarrhea, increased blood-fat levels	Improved fertility

3. Avoid supplements labeled "high-potency" or "therapeutic." These products typically contain levels of vitamins and minerals that greatly exceed the RDA and may be hazardous (see "Supplement Hazards" below).

4. Avoid supplements that contain nonessential substances. "Vitamin B_{15}," inositol, PABA, rutin, bioflavonoids, and rose hips are all nonessential nutrients that have not been proven beneficial to health. Instead, such substances needlessly add to the price of protecting your well-being.

5. Choose a supplement based on its contents and not on a higher price. Generic brands of supplements are comparable in quality to higher-price brands (make sure the supplement meets guideline 1). Also, such words as "natural" or "organic" do not indicate a better source of vitamin or mineral. In some cases, the synthetic vitamin is better absorbed than the naturally occurring form of the vitamin.

6. Choose a supplement in tablet form. Gimmicks like "timed-release" or "effervescent" (dissolves in water like an Alka-Seltzer) are not worth the additional expense. Timed-release vitamin and mineral supplements do not have an advantage over the standard tablet. Vitamins and minerals need food for absorption into the body, and with timed-release supplements some vitamin and/or mineral may pass through unabsorbed. Effervescent supplements do show better absorption for riboflavin, a B vitamin, when compared with a standard tablet. However, for most vitamins, the absorption difference is insignificant compared with absorption from a standard tablet, making the cost a little tough to swallow.

SUPPLEMENT HAZARDS

It's almost an instinctual behavior. If some vitamin or mineral is optimal for health and performance, people think more must be better for health and performance. I'll be honest with you; I have felt the same. But when I remove the mystique that surrounds vitamins and minerals, logical reasons for taking additional amounts of these nutrients disappear.

When your body has a sufficient amount of a particular vitamin or mineral, additional amounts do not enhance the function of that nutrient. Instead, the vitamin or mineral overload must be

Table 5-9 *MEGADOSE CAUTIONS: THOSE WHO SHOULD BEWARE*

The hazards of vitamin overdosing are real for everyone. Some individuals in certain situations, however, are at greater risk of suffering from the perils of vitamin intoxication.

Vitamin	Condition	Consequences
Vitamin A	Pregnancy	Risks birth defects
Niacin (B_3)	Diabetes	Aggravates symptoms
	Heart disease	Can cause arrhythmias
Vitamin B_6	Breastfeeding	May inhibit milk production
Folate	Epilepsy	Interferes with drug treatment
Vitamin C	Diabetes	Interferes with urine tests
	Kidney stones	Precipitates stones in urinary tract
	Pregnancy	Can cause rebound scurvy in newborns
	Vegetarian	Destroys vitamin B_{12} in food—a vitamin which is absent in strict vegetarian diets
Vitamin D	Kidney stones	Precipitates stones
Vitamin E	Heart disease	Can cause blood-fat levels to increase; interferes with medication for anticoagulation

dealt with by your body. Either the excess is excreted in the urine (usually the water-soluble vitamins and some minerals—sodium, potassium) or it is stored in the body, running the risk of toxic side effects (fat-soluble vitamins and some minerals—selenium, iron, zinc, copper).

The consequences of vitamin or mineral overdosing can be insignificant (brightly colored and expensive urine is all you get from too much riboflavin). But many vitamins and minerals in excess result in dangerous, if not deadly, consequences. Vitamin and mineral overdoses may also mask a medical disorder, interfere with the body's use of another nutrient, or precipitate a nutritional deficiency.

Keep in mind that vitamins and minerals can act like strong drugs when they are taken in amounts that exceed their duties as essential nutrients. While levels that cause toxic side effects vary for each particular vitamin and mineral, ten times the RDA for any given nutrient is considered megadosing and ill-advised. Perhaps you'll consider a rather simple piece of advice: I always say if Mother Nature intended us to consume large amounts of vitamins and minerals, her fruits, vegetables, grains, and other unprocessed foods would have more in them.

Vitamin and mineral overdosing hazards are real but can easily be avoided if you choose a supplement wisely and use it when it's appropriate. Check Tables 5-8 and 5-9 for megadosing hazards and to find out who is at particular risk for supplement overdose side effects.

PART TWO

POWER-EATING PLAN

CHAPTER 6

EATING MANAGEMENT

Your day starts at a hectic pace: wake-up alarm, rapid-fire dressing, perhaps dealing with the kids, morning commute, staff meeting at nine, and on and on. This is what I call the "A.M. mayhem." No wonder you skip breakfast and have no idea what you will eat for lunch, let alone where. As for dinner, it's a distant mystery. Your fast-paced schedule demands stamina as well as high-quality performance, yet your eating habits doom you to failure.

In a sense, the challenges of home and workplace today demand that you perform at the same level as a professional athlete. Like the marathon runner, you are continually attempting to go further, do more, and in less time. Isn't that what success is today—doing more in less time? Conquering this hectic pace is impossible unless you consume the right fuels at the right time.

From earlier chapters, you now know the basics of high-performance eating set forth in the 60-15-25 Power Diet—the carbohydrate, protein, and fat calorie balance for success. Due to your urgent schedule, "marathon" days happen frequently, and fitting in power meals and snacks can provide the staying power you need to keep going. Your brain requires a constant supply of nutrients—carbohydrates for energy and protein, vitamins, and minerals for sharp functioning. Your muscles also require this same flow of energizing nutrition.

In this and the following chapters, you will select your own Power Eating Strategies. First, check on your present eating style by taking my Power Foods Quiz, and identify trouble spots that may be sapping your performance. Then, my simple, ten-step Power-Eating Guide puts the Power Diet to work for you. You will have eating strategies and menus you can use when traveling, dining out, meeting erratic work schedules, and during long business meetings. You will have a Power-Eating Plan tailored to harness the ultimate performance food—carbohydrate—for optimum day-to-day stamina and performance.

EATING FOR PERFORMANCE

You manage your time to optimize your success—at work, at home, and in fitness activities. Now think of managing your eating for optimal performance, too. What you eat for lunch, for example, can determine your energy levels during the long afternoon at the office. If you miss a meal, what you eat next, and when, can determine your fatigue level—mentally and physically—for the balance of that day. More on these and other Power Eating guidelines later in this chapter, but first you must evaluate your present eating style. You can do that with my Power Foods Quiz.

Do you get enough energizing carbohydrate and power protein, along with crucial vitamins and minerals, for top performance? Are your eating habits and calorie balance adding to or subtracting from your health and vitality? First compare your score for each section, then your total quiz score, with my Power Diet standards to get a rating for your eating habits. (For more detail, check with the explanation for individual questions that follows the test.)

BEFORE YOU TAKE THE QUIZ

Because these questions focus on key aspects of what you eat and when you eat it over three consecutive days, your quiz results will be most useful if you record everything you eat at the time rather than estimate the amounts and frequency as you take the quiz. Keep track of snacks, beverages, seasonings, how foods were prepared, and precise size of servings. Don't change your eating habits before you take this quiz; an accurate record of your usual diet is best. It will be helpful if you read over the quiz at least three days before you take it to see what you'll be asked.

THE POWER FOODS QUIZ

Read each question and review your diary, then circle the appropriate answer. If you're asked for the average number of servings per day, divide the total number of servings consumed in the three days by three. Of course, estimate servings when you're not sure, but try to be realistic about it. The purpose is to analyze the real you and aim for improvement, not necessarily perfection. (Quiz developed by Liz Applegate, Ph.D., and Judith Stern, Sc.D., R.D.)

Section 1: Power Diet
Possible Points: 70

Performance Carbohydrates
1. How many servings of grain products did you eat daily? (1 serving = 1 slice of bread, ½ bagel or a muffin, ½ cup cooked grain; do not include high-fat, high-sugar biscuits, croissants, cookies, cakes, and the like.)
a. 6 or more (5 points)
b. 4 to 5 (4 points)
c. 2 to 3 (2 points)
d. 1 (1 point)
e. None (0 points)

2. What type of bread (including rolls, muffins, and such) do you usually eat?

a. Whole-wheat, rye, oat, or multigrain(4 points)

b. White or partial whole-wheat (2 points)

3. How many servings of oat bran, rice bran, or wheat bran products did you average daily? (1 serving = 1 cup cooked oatmeal or oat bran.)

a. 2 or more (3 points)

b. 1 (2 points)

c. ½ (1 point)

d. None (0 points)

4. How many servings of leafy green vegetables did you eat daily? (1 serving = 1 cup raw or ½ cup cooked: kale, collard greens, spinach, broccoli, dark-green leaf lettuce.)

a. 2 or more (5 points)

b. 1 (4 points)

c. ½ (3 points)

d. None (−1 point)

5. How many times during the three-day period did you eat legumes or legume products: tofu; kidney, pinto, or garbanzo beans; soybeans; lentils; split peas?

a. 3 or more (4 points)

b. 2 (3 points)

c. 1 (2 points)

d. None (0 points)

6. How many servings of orange-yellow vegetables or fruits did you eat during the three days? (1 serving = ½ cup cooked, 1 cup raw, ½ cup juice: winter squash, pumpkin, carrot, melon, peach, apricot.)

a. 3 or more (5 points)

b. 2 (3 points)

c. 1 (2 points)

d. None (0 points)

7. How many servings of citrus fruits, strawberries, or green peppers did you eat during the three days? (1 serving = 1 whole, ½ cup juice, 1 cup raw.)

a. 3 or more (4 points)

b. 2 (3 points)
c. 1 (2 points)
d. None (0 points)

8. How many servings of cruciferous vegetables did you eat during the three days? (1 serving = ½ cup cooked or 1 cup raw: broccoli, cauliflower, cabbage, brussels sprouts, bok choy, turnip, rutabaga, kale.)
a. 3 or more (4 points)
b. 2 (3 points)
c. 1 (2 points)
d. None (0 points)

Power Protein

9. How many servings of milk, yogurt, cheese, tofu, or soy-milk product did you have daily? If you're using cream or half-and-half, don't count these. (1 serving = 1 cup milk, yogurt; 1 ounce cheese.)
a. 3 or more (5 points)
b. 2 (4 points)
c. 1 (3 points)
d. None (−1 point)

10. How many servings of meat, fish, or poultry did you eat daily? (1 serving = 3 ounces cooked, about the size of a deck of playing cards.)
a. More than 2 servings (−1 point)
b. 1 to 2 (2 points)
c. None (0 points)

High-Performance Fat

11. What do you usually spread on your bread, toast, rolls, or muffins?
a. Butter, cream cheese, mayonnaise (−2 points)
b. Margarine (0 points)
c. Jam, mustard (2 points)
d. Fruit spread or nothing (4 points)

12. What type of dairy products do you usually eat?
a. Half-and-half, nondairy creamer (−3 points)
b. Whole milk (−1 point)

c. 2% milk (2 points)

d. 1% milk (3 points)

e. Nonfat or skim milk (4 points)

13. During the three days, how many times did you eat processed meats (bacon, luncheon meats, sausage, salami)?

a. 3 or more (−3 points)

b. 2 (−2 points)

c. 1 (1 point)

d. None (3 points)

14. Did you remove skin from poultry and trim visible fat from meats?

a. Yes (4 points)

b. No (−2 points)

15. How many egg yolks did you consume during the three-day period (in cooking or eaten as an egg dish)?

a. 3 or more (−1 point)

b. 2 (0 points)

c. 1 (1 point)

d. None (3 points)

16. When preparing meals or eating out, how many times during the three days were foods cooked in oil (fried), sautéed in butter or margarine, or prepared with cream sauce?

a. 5 or more (−2 points)

b. 3 to 4 (−1 point)

c. 1 to 2 (0 points)

d. none (3 points)

17. Over three days, how many times did you eat snack crackers, chips, or baked goods that contained butter, lard, hydrogenated vegetable fat, coconut oil, or palm oil?

a. 5 or more (−3 points)

b. 3 to 4 (0 points)

c. 1 to 2 (2 points)

d. none (4 points)

18. What type of dressing did you usually put on your salad?

a. Regular salad dressing or oil and vinegar (−1 point)

b. Reduced calorie (i.e., low-fat) dressing (3 points)
c. Lemon juice, tomato juice, nonfat bottled dressings, vinegar, or none (4 points)

Section 2: Diet Extras
Possible Points: 19

19. What seasonings did you typically add to foods?
a. Garlic, herbs, lemon juice, vinegar, no-salt spices (4 points)
b. Salt substitute, mustard (3 points)
c. Soy sauce, garlic or onion salt, teriyaki sauce, pickle relish (1 point)
d. Salt (−1 point)

20. Over the three-day period, how many alcoholic drinks did you average? (1 serving = 12 ounces beer, 4 ounces wine, or 1 ounce liquor.)
a. 2 or more (−5 points)
b. 1 (−1 point)
c. None (4 points)

21. What beverage did you drink most frequently with meals or snacks?
a. Water, mineral water, soda water, or skim milk (4 points)
b. Fruit juice (3 points)
c. Diet soda (1 point)
d. Fruit drink, soda, coffee, or tea (0 points)

22. How many servings of caffeine-containing beverages did you drink daily? (1 serving = 6 ounces coffee, 10 ounces tea, 16 ounces soda.)
a. 3 or more (−2 points)
b. 2 (0 points)
c. 1 (1 point)
d. None (3 points)

23. How many times did you eat high-sugar, high-calorie foods (pie, cake, candy, chocolate, cookies, ice cream)?
a. 3 or more (−2 points)
b. 2 (0 points)
c. 1 (2 points)
d. None (4 points)

Section 3: Eating Style
Possible Points: 21

24. How many times did you skip a regular meal during the three days?

a. Not at all (5 points)

b. 1 time (2 points)

c. 2 times (0 points)

d. 3 or more times (−2 points)

25. If you skipped a meal, did you snack lightly before your next meal?

a. Yes (2 points)

b. No (0 points)

26. Did you consistently plan at least 30 minutes before-hand what and when you would be eating?

a. Always (5 points)

b. Most often (3 points)

c. Rarely (0 points)

d. Never (−3 points)

27. How many meals did you plan and shop for ahead of time during the three-day period?

a. 5 or more meals (5 points)

b. 3 to 4 meals (3 points)

c. 1 to 2 meals (0 points)

d. None (−2 points)

28. How often during the three-day period did you spon-taneously get something that you felt wasn't a good food choice to eat as a pick-me-up?

a. Not at all (4 points)

b. 1 or 2 times (2 points)

c. 3 times (0 points)

d. 4 or more times (−2 points)

Section 4: Weight Control
Possible Points: 15

29. Are you ten or more pounds over the weight you would like to be?

a. Yes (0 points)

b. No (6 points)

30. Have you lost and then regained ten or more pounds in the past one to two years?

a. Yes (-2 points)

b. No (5 points)

31. Do you reward yourself for doing a job or completing a task with an edible treat of some kind?

a. Frequently (-3 points)

b. Rarely (0 points)

c. Never (4 points)

Your Total Quiz Score:

How did you do? Maximum possible points: 125. Your overall score gives you a general idea of whether your diet is in good shape or needs work.

Over 100 points: Excellent! You're probably eating the Power Diet already. Check "Identify Your Trouble Spots" for a little fine-tuning.

85 to 100 points: Good job. You're eating for good health. Make a few changes to eat for success. Check your problem areas in the next section for some suggestions.

65 to 84 points: Fair. Your diet needs some work—go over each section of the test and see what changes will get you on track with Power Eating.

Less than 65 points: You're running on three cylinders. Your potential for improvement will astound you. Begin by carefully reviewing the recommendations in the next section, along with the Power-Eating Plan, for a fresh start. Evaluate your shopping habits and eating style by comparing them with guidelines from the next three chapters.

IDENTIFY YOUR TROUBLE SPOTS

Now that you know how your diet rates overall, use your score on individual sections of the Power Foods Quiz to pinpoint potential weak spots. Compare your score for each section with the numbers below to help you hone in on danger areas. Also, if you check your score on individual questions or sets of questions, you can fine-tune your diet using the suggestions below.

You may find it helpful to take the quiz again in about two months to see how the changes you made are working for you. I frequently take the test myself (often just Section 1) to make sure my Power Eating stays on track.

Section 1: Power Diet. This section gives you an idea of how close you are to eating the Power Diet, that is, 60 percent of your calories from carbs, 15 percent from protein, and 25 percent from fat. While a computerized diet analysis will give exact numbers, your score on this section is a good indication of how you are doing.

If you scored over 56 points (70 points maximum) on this section, you're probably eating within the Power Diet guidelines. If under 56 points, check specific questions for suggestions.

Questions 1 through 8: Performance Carbohydrates. Eating more carbohydrate-rich foods in the place of high-fat food choices is basic to your Power Diet. For Question 1, six or more servings of grain products like bread, cereal, rice, and potatoes is crucial if you are to get enough energizing carbs each day. These foods also supply many vitamins and minerals associated with energy metabolism. Whole-grain products (Question 2) supply fiber, zinc, magnesium, vitamin E, and vitamin B_6, in addition to the B vitamins and iron found in enriched grain products. Fiber and additional nutrients are supplied by oat and other bran products as well as green leafy vegetables (Questions 3 and 4).

Beans (kidney beans, garbanzos, and soybeans) are loaded with carbohydrates while supplying some excellent quality protein, especially if eaten with rice, pasta, or other grain foods (Question 5). Questions 6, 7, and 8 zero in on your intake of the standout vitamins and minerals as well as carbohydrates. Try to eat at least one serving of vitamin C-rich fruit or vegetables along with a serving of cruciferous vegetables and green leafy vegetables each day for maximum nutrition.

Questions 9 and 10: Power Protein. To get the protein you need to match your active lifestyle, eat two to three servings of low-fat or nonfat dairy products or soy-based foods daily, along with one or two 3-ounce servings of lean meat, fish, or poultry. If you get your protein from beans and grains, then eat the equivalent of ½ cup cooked beans with approximately 1 cup cooked grains in place of a meat or fish serving. Dairy products supply the calcium and riboflavin your body needs for stamina and strength. If you avoid dairy products, look to soy-based foods like soy milk as a replacement. Also, remember that meats are a great source of iron and zinc. Green leafy vegetables, along with cooked beans, can act as an alternate source of these minerals if you abstain from meat. (Check Tables 3-3 and 3-4 on pages 95 and 98 for more Power Protein suggestions.)

Questions 11 through 18: High-Performance Fats. As you know from chapter 4, you need fat for optimal health, but too much or the wrong type of fat can endanger your performance and well-being. If you scored a total of 19 points or more for these questions (25 maximum), then your fat intake is probably in the neighborhood of 25 percent of total calories. But if you scored less than 19 points, review each question to find your trouble spots. Questions 11 and 12 test your saturated fat intake, which, as you also know from chapter 4, may elevate your blood cholesterol levels. Processed meats (Question 13) also pack extra saturated fat and sodium. You're better off avoiding these meats or selecting lower-fat versions, like lean ham or roasted turkey and chicken lunch meats.

Removing skin from poultry and limiting your egg yolk intake to two per week (Questions 14 and 15) are good ways to keep fat and cholesterol intake down. This allows more room for energizing carbs, like an extra serving of rice or potatoes, at your meal. Preparing foods in nonstick pans without the use of added fats such as oils, butter, and lard (Question 16) also helps lower fat calories to the desired 25 percent. Many snack foods prepared with hydrogenated vegetable oils contain at least 30 to 50 percent fat calories. Instead of chips and snack crackers, munch on pretzels, air-popped popcorn, and rice cakes for less fat and more carbs. Dressing your salads with low-calorie salad dressings (Question 18) or, better yet, lemon juice and/or vinegar will help you shave fat calories without sacrificing taste. You may also find that a mild salsa on mixed greens is a very tasty substitute for high-fat salad dressings.

After evaluating your response to these questions, if you feel you could improve some, take this portion of the quiz over again in a month or two. (Check "Strategies for Conquering the Fat

Issue" on page 136 for more suggestions on controlling the amount of fat in your diet.) You'll find that once you identify the high-fat foods you typically eat, lowering fat intake and boosting carbohydrate calories for increased stamina will be a cinch.

Section 2: Diet Extras. This section looks at the little extras in your diet, like salt, alcohol, sugar, and caffeine. If you scored below 15 points (19 maximum), scan your food diary for extras that can sap your performance.

Question 19. A high sodium intake is linked to high blood pressure, a risk factor for heart disease. When possible, use herbs, vinegars, and mustards instead of salt or salt-containing seasonings (some salt substitutes actually contain sodium). Also, look at your responses to Questions 13 and 17. Processed meats and snack foods can add substantially to your sodium intake.

Question 20. Alcohol is best avoided, since this substance offers nothing but calories. Used in excess, alcohol depletes your body of precious minerals and B vitamins. If your body's ability to process alcohol is exceeded (usually when more than one or two drinks are consumed in an hour), then carbohydrate and protein metabolisms are also negatively affected.

Question 21. When choosing a beverage other than water, reach for fluids that have some nutritional punch. Skim milk and fruit juices supply vitamins and minerals (milk is also a great source of quality protein). If you are watching your weight, limit fruit juices as a thirst quencher since they do contain 60 calories per ½-cup serving. Sodas and fruit drinks (as opposed to juices) are high in sugar and empty calories.

Questions 21 and 22. Caffeine-containing beverages should be consumed in moderation, if at all. Excessive caffeine intake can cause nervousness, insomnia, and increased body-water losses, leaving you feeling and performing at less than 100 percent.

Question 23. Sugary foods pack calories but few nutrients. Sweets also detract from your daily intake of energizing complex carbs like potatoes, grains, and cereals. Use the tips in "Eat Sweets the Right Way" on page 79 to help limit your sugar intake. By reducing sugar in your diet, you make room for other foods packed with power nutrients.

Section 3: Eating Style. Here you focus on eating habits that may be detracting from your day-to-day performance. If you scored below 16 points for this section (maximum of 21 points), you need to fine-tune your eating style to maximize your performance.

Questions 24 through 28. When you skip a meal (Question 24), your body loses out on carbs needed for stamina as well as power nutrients, protein, vitamins, and minerals. Missing breakfast, for example, can mean less efficient work in the late morning hours and poor performance during a noon workout. Irregular eating may also interfere with controlling body weight. If skipping a meal is unavoidable, snack lightly on high-carbohydrate foods to reinforce your energy levels and to keep yourself from overeating at the next meal (Question 25).

Another essential for maintaining top energy levels is knowing what and when you will be eating (Questions 26 and 27). A little planning helps you to avoid splurging—that is, eating foods you know are high in fat and low on energizing carbs. If you plan on having a late dinner, for instance, snack lightly in the afternoon to keep the hungries away.

When you start to lag, avoid reaching for a pick-me-up that is low in power nutrients. It can only rob you of strength for the job at hand (Question 28).

Section 4: Weight Control. These questions examine weight maintenance and behavior. If you scored less than 11 points for these three questions (maximum points: 15), then weight control may be a factor in your under-par health and performance.

Questions 29 through 31. Being overweight (Question 29) can make simple activities like lifting, walking, or just getting into your car difficult. Extra pounds can also limit your ability to exercise and detract from your health. Obese people are at greater risk for heart disease and certain types of cancer. The next chapter will help you find your ideal calorie balance and get control of your weight.

Weight yo-yoing—losing and regaining weight—can put you on a roller coaster to poor health and performance (Question 31). It slows your metabolism, can lead to greater fat gain, and makes each successive attempt at weight loss more difficult. Even if you gain and lose the "same" ten pounds, weight cycling can retard your performance by increasing your desire for high-fat foods.

Behavior that contributes to weight gain often centers around the use of food as a reward (Question 31). If you find yourself having treats in reward for a day's work or just because you deserve something, turn to "Dining-Out Tactics" on page 231 for some tips on how to reward yourself with positive results.

TRY AGAIN

After you have identified your trouble spots and made solid efforts to smooth the rough edges of your diet, take the quiz again. Wait about eight weeks or so, giving the changes a chance to become part of your daily routine, before you take the entire quiz. You may find that quizzing yourself periodically on the Power Diet section (Section 1) is a good way to keep your eating skills finely tuned.

POWER-EATING GUIDE: TEN STEPS TO FOLLOW DAILY TO MAINTAIN YOUR COMPETITIVE EDGE

You analyzed your diet and found its weak spots—now you are on your way to eating for power. Since today's home, workplace, and fitness challenges demand that you perform, in a sense, at a level comparable to that of a professional athlete, you need a simple plan to be sure you get the right fuel at the right time. My Power-Eating Guide provides simple steps that guarantee your success. These guidelines are the basis for the Power Diet, and they incorporate what you already know about Power Eating. Follow these ten steps daily and get ready for success!

1. Eat breakfast. Of course, you have heard this before, but this time think about eating breakfast regularly as a performance booster. Studies show that missing breakfast can undercut reading skills, memory, and the ability to concentrate. Researchers find a poorer attitude among schoolchildren who miss breakfast. If this carries over to adults, it may help explain why you may sometimes have an "attitude problem" at work. It can also explain why you sometimes work less efficiently in the late morning hours.

Try a breakfast of whole-grain cereal, skim milk, and fruit for a dose of complex carbohydrates that will cause a slow and steady release of glucose into your bloodstream. This flow of energy over a few hours feeds your brain and muscles with needed energy. Selecting nutritious foods like fruit, whole-grain breads, and cereals over "empty foods" (doughnuts and pastries) gives your body the vitamins and minerals it needs to perform.

2. Have a power snack to recover quickly from a missed meal. If you can't avoid missing breakfast on occasion, or if you miss lunch, don't hold off until your next meal to "make up" for lost calories. Instead, have a snack to power yourself into action until your next meal. Don't worry about spoiling your appetite; your body needs nourishment to overcome feelings of low energy.

Aim for high-carbohydrate snacks with minimal fat and protein, in the range of 200 to 300 calories—a sliced bagel topped with one ounce of mozzarella cheese and a can of vegetable juice, or a carton of low-fat yogurt with one cup fresh fruit salad, for example. This type of mini-meal provides needed carbohydrates for energy.

3. Lunch lightly and pace yourself. Overeating at lunch can make for a sluggish performance in midafternoon. Behavior researchers report that scores on mental acuity tests were lower in those subjects fed large lunches (1,000-plus calories). Sluggishness and sleepiness were more common in subjects who were used to eating large midday meals.

Avoid overeating by planning your day's meals. *Knowing the when and where of your lunch and dinner can keep you from splurging.* If mealtime is delayed, snack lightly on high-carbohydrate foods, such as unbuttered popcorn and whole-grain bread. This will help curb a ravenous appetite and prevent "treating" yourself to a large meal.

Also, pace your eating at meals. It takes about 20 minutes for your brain to get the signal that your stomach has had enough. That's why rapid eating leads to greater calorie intake at mealtime.

4. Include some protein at lunch. True, carbohydrates are the quickest energy source, but unless they are balanced with protein at the midday meal, you may feel a bit sluggish. Truly high-carbohydrate meals, such as a bread-and-fruit combination, can increase the brain's level of serotonin, a chemical responsible for sleepiness and calmness. Protein, on the other hand, increases alertness by changing the levels of brain chemicals called catecholamines.

While this food/mood link is still controversial, a low-fat, high-protein, low-calorie lunch is your best bet for afternoon efficiency. Negative mood changes have been linked to eating high-carbohydrate lunches. (Since alertness peaks in the morning, this is not true of a high-carbohydrate breakfast.)

Your noontime meal should include a solid protein source—lean meat, fish, low-fat cheese, milk, egg, or tofu/grain dish. Balance this with complex carbohydrates—breads, fruits, vegetables—for a supply of glucose energy.

5. Eat every three to four hours to keep energy flowing. It's a fact: A midafternoon snack invigorates your mind. Tests show that individuals, when fed a snack 15 minutes before comparing skills of memory, alertness, math problem solving, and reading, performed better than those fed nothing before testing, even though both groups had eaten breakfast and lunch. Snacking improved memory and alertness scores by 15 to 20 percent. Current research shows that the increase in blood sugar from a snack gives the brain an energy boost which lasts a few hours.

If you find yourself lagging at midmorning or in the afternoon, try a light snack rich in carbohydrate. Adding snacks to your daily eating routine shouldn't lead to weight gain if you control calories at other meals. In fact, some studies show that eating five to six times a day helps in weight control, as opposed to eating one or two meals daily.

Snack on healthful between-meal choices such as whole-grain crackers, unsalted pretzels, plain popcorn, fruit and fruit juices, vegetable sticks, and vegetable juices. Check vending machines for healthful snacks (see "Workday Lunching Plan" on page 241), useful especially while on the road and in other difficult-to-deal-with eating locations.

6. Aim for regular mealtimes. Consistent mealtimes make for predictable performance. Try to eat breakfast, lunch, dinner, and snacks at the same time each day. Such a routine reinforces moderate-sized, well-planned meals and snacks. Slipping into a sporadic eating schedule, on the other hand, puts you on a performance roller coaster. Long stretches without eating, and then overeating, can mean sluggish performance when you can least afford it.

7. Include complex carbohydrates in every meal and snack. Supply your brain with a steady flow of energy from complex carbohydrates. Unlike fat and protein, complex carbs start entering the bloodstream almost immediately. Remember that because complex carbohydrates are made from linked sugar units, they break down more slowly than simple sugars, resulting in a steady release of glucose into your system.

Use hot or cold cereals, muffins, bagels, breads, or fruit at breakfast. Pasta, rice, potatoes, vegetables, and cooked beans are just a few lunch and dinner suggestions. Snack on traditional high-carbohydrate foods such as crackers, popcorn, pretzels, and fruit. You may want to try a cold baked potato, rice tossed with raisins and cinnamon, or low-sugar breakfast cereal bits in a bag for snacking variety.

8. Keep stamina-enhancing foods on hand. Stow some emergency stamina-sustaining foods at work or in your carry bag for a quick snack or meal add-on. Keeping power foods within reach prevents productivity dips due to missed or delayed meals. Your gym bag, glove compartment, desk drawer, and, of course, your briefcase make good storage spots for small cans of fruit or vegetable juices, dried fruit, small packages of whole-grain crackers, rice cakes, or fruit and nut mix.

9. Curb your caffeine intake. While a cup of coffee, strong tea, or caffeine-containing soft drink may pick you up from a midmorning or late-afternoon energy dip, too much caffeine can deplete your energy. Excessive amounts of caffeine (for most people, about five cups of coffee a day or the equivalent) can make you nervous and restless and make it difficult for you to fall asleep as well (see chapter 1 for more about caffeine).

Avoid excessive coffee drinking, particularly on days when you're listless, such as after a poor night's sleep. Instead, stick to your eating plan and choose your favorite revitalizing foods: maybe crunchy vegetable sticks or soda water mixed with fruit juice, along with a good body stretch or a brief walk.

10. Keep your sweet tooth under control. Resist that craving for a candy bar or sugary soda as an energy pick-me-up. You may feel you're getting a lift, but you're really not doing much for your body nutritionally, and you may actually feel sluggish after a high-sugar snack due to changes it causes in brain chemistry.

Most high-sugar snacks are loaded with fat and are low in power nutrients. Eating a well-balanced diet, with an occasional sweet, is best to keep you performing at peak levels. If you must indulge in sweetened goodies, eat them during or right after a meal. The simple sugars from sweets will mix in your stomach with the contents of your entire meal, causing a slower release of sugar into your bloodstream. Waiting until mealtime to eat sweets also helps to limit consumption of simple sugars.

CHAPTER **7**

FINDING YOUR CALORIE BALANCE

A crucial part of your Power-Eating Plan is to achieve a balance between the calories you eat and the calories your body burns. Unless you have that balance, your health and your performance are at risk. The excess energy from too many calories is stored as fat; too few calories, on the other hand, leaves your energy stores drained, resulting in chronic fatigue and susceptibility to illness and injury.

In previous chapters, you saw that carbohydrates, protein, and fat supply you with energy needed for stamina at work and during exercise. You also know that the Power Diet of 60-15-25 (see "The Power Diet Solution" on page 135) is the optimal distribution of calories from carbohydrate, protein, and fat. But how many calories do you need each day to stay in balance? How do you know if you're eating too much or too little?

This chapter provides the answer. It tells you:

- ☐ How many calories you need for day-to-day stamina.
- ☐ How to beat a slow metabolism.
- ☐ The difference between the way your body handles fat calories and carbohydrate calories.
- ☐ The shape of your body in terms of acceptable fat distribution.
- ☐ Whether you should lose or gain weight—or perhaps even stop participating in the great American pastime of worrying about your weight.

You will also read about the hazards of too few calories—running on empty—as well as the concerns of being overweight. Finally, I outline ten steps essential to controlling your weight for a lifetime and give you tips on how to choose a weight-loss program and succeed at it.

CALORIES: HOW MANY ARE YOU BURNING?

You can't see calories or taste them, but you can feel calories. From a chemist's point of view, a calorie is a measure of heat. For example, 100 calories—about the number in two sugar cookies—is the amount of heat needed to convert a quart of ice into boiling water. We laymen look at a calorie differently. To us, a calorie represents food's energy that runs our basic bodily functions—breathing, metabolism, circulation—plus any voluntary physical activity we perform.

The number of calories in any food can be determined easily. Every gram of both protein and carbohydrate contains four calories, while fat contains nine calories per gram. Knowing this, you can compute the calories in all the foods you eat. Most packaged foods and beverages already have the number of calories listed on the package label, so there is no need for you to do the calculation.

The number of calories in a food (100 calories in a banana, for example) represents the amount of energy released from the food when your body "burns" it (more accurately—the energy released when the chemical bonds from carbohydrate, protein, and fat are broken during metabolism). In theory, a calorie is a calorie is a calorie; that is, regardless of where the calorie comes from (protein, carbohydrate, or fat), your body uses it the same way. But when it comes to fat calories, this may not be the case.

In chapter 2, I pointed out that your body tends to treat fat calories more efficiently than carbohydrate or protein calories. Many studies link obesity to a high-fat diet rather than simply a diet with too many calories. This suggests that the body can store or convert fat calories to body fat more easily than it can store or convert carbohydrate or protein calories to fat. Other studies show that even when calorie intake is low, a high proportion of fat in the diet can still mean production of body fat. This "fattening" action of dietary fat is still another reason to eat the 60-15-25 Power Diet.

BALANCING YOUR ENERGY EQUATION

As a person interested in maximizing your performance—on the job, at home, and in the gym—you want to know how many calories you need to stay energized without risking excess weight gain. Everyone has a personal calorie requirement for balancing the number of calories taken in from food with the number of calories the body ordinarily burns each day.

Your energy equation is yours alone. The number of calories you burn depends upon your body weight, gender, age, activity level, and whether you smoke or use caffeinated drinks, among other factors. You can easily figure your calorie needs by following a few steps.

For starters, most of your energy needs are dictated by the amount you need to support life's essentials—heartbeat, breathing, digestion, brain functions—your basal metabolic rate (BMR). It accounts for 60 to 75 percent of your daily calorie consumption. Men, for example, need more calories than women do because they have more metabolically active muscle mass. Women, on the other hand, have more of the metabolically sluggish component—fat.

And older people need fewer calories than younger folks because metabolism slows after age 20. The amount of slowdown is somewhere around 2 percent every ten years. Thus, a

70-year-old man needs about ten percent fewer calories to support basal metabolism than he did when he was 20.

You can work out your own numbers for BMR. Adult men require approximately 11 calories per day for every pound of body weight, and women need 10. To figure your basal energy needs, multiply your body weight by the appropriate number. For example, I weigh 115 pounds, so my basal metabolic rate is: 115 pounds times 10 calories/pound equals 1,150 calories needed per day.

If I were to lounge around all day and do absolutely nothing, I would still need 1,150 calories just to maintain my calorie balance (and keep my weight in balance). But when I do anything more than just lie still, I require even more calories, above and beyond my BMR. I expend calories when I eat food (yes, digestion requires calories, but unfortunately, not enough to be called exercise). Any type of activity—sitting, standing, walking, jogging, swimming, or cycling, for example—burns additional calories.

The amount of energy you need to manage foods is quite small—about 5 percent or less of your total calorie intake. You can ignore figuring this into your energy balance equation because, more than likely, there is at least a 5 percent error in calculating the calories needed for basal functions and for activity.

Caloric needs for physical activity, on the other hand, can be quite extensive, and this is where you need to make a reasonable estimate of how "calorically busy" your day is. A quick and easy method to roughly figure your daily caloric need is to assign yourself an activity level that describes your overall calorie expenditure for your daily business (work, home life, and exercise).

There are four different levels of activity. Each represents additional calories your body requires, expressed as a percentage of your basal metabolic rate. This means that if you fit into the moderate category, for example, you burn an additional 70 percent above your basal energy needs during the day for activity. Check Table 7-1 for your activity level.

So using myself as an example, my BMR is 1,150 calories per day and my activity level is strenuous (between my job, which

Table 7-1 *BASAL METABOLIC RATE (BMR) FOR FOUR LEVELS OF ACTIVITY*

Activity Level	Description	Additional % of BMR
Sedentary	Sitting job (desk worker), little or no regular exercise	30–50
Light	Standing job (teacher), some regular exercise (walking)	55–65
Moderate	Active job with a lot of movement (day care), regular exercise (3 to 4 times per week, 30 to 40 minutes)	65–70
Strenuous	Labor job (lifting, construction), regular exercise (4 times per week, 40 minutes)	75–100

SOURCE: Adapted from E. N. Whitney et al., *Understanding Nutrition,* 5th ed. (St. Paul, Minn.: West Publishing Co., 1990).

involves some sitting and standing, and about two hours of endurance exercise daily). I need an additional 80 percent of my BMR for activity: 1,150 plus 80 percent of 1,150 (920) equals 2,070 calories needed per day.

Figure out your calorie needs for the day. The number you arrive at is fairly close to your actual calorie requirement. Only a special laboratory could determine it more precisely. Your goal now is to stay in balance with this number of calories. Use eating strategies from the next chapters to compose menus that will keep you in calorie balance and give you day-long stamina.

As you know, if you take in more calories than you burn, your body must store the extras as body fat. While many individuals may hate their bodies for this energy efficiency, it is a long-standing survival mechanism from our caveman ancestors, who had to survive during times of little food. In addition to storing extra calories as fat, some people must eat fewer calories than expected to stay in energy balance. What these people face are the woes of a very efficient calorie utilization, that is, a low BMR.

DO YOU HAVE A LOW METABOLISM?

After calculating your calorie needs, your fears are reconfirmed—you believe you are already eating less than the calculations indicate you need. Based on the equations, you should be able to consume another couple of hundred calories daily, but you know if you were to do that you'd gain weight. What gives? You may be suffering from a slow metabolism, a BMR lower than expected. This doesn't mean your body is in slow motion, but rather, your basal metabolism is energy efficient. Like it or not, yours is actually a more finely tuned machine that requires less energy than most.

A low metabolism may just be a family trait. Many studies show a genetic factor in caloric expenditure. Consider your other family members—are they battling overweight despite low calorie intake? Besides genetics, other factors may change your metabolism rate. For instance, taking in too few calories may trigger your body's natural survival instincts and lower your BMR, so you require even fewer calories. People who diet frequently often trigger this decrease in their metabolism rate, creating even more of a challenge for themselves in their weight-loss endeavors. Also, people who exercise regularly and cut back on their calorie intake to stay slim may slow down their metabolism (more on this in "Running on Empty" later in this chapter).

YOUR BODY: LEARN TO LIKE IT

More than likely, you have been unhappy with your body at one time or another—its shape, its weight, or both. Perhaps you feel you should lose five or ten pounds or that your thighs are too thick. You're not alone. Most of us feel that our bodies could look a little better. After all, some 34 million Americans are obese, risking heart disease, cancer, and other ailments because of it. But on the other hand, many of us have unreal expectations of what our bodies could look like and how much weight we could lose.

For starters, many people are obsessed with achieving a certain "look." Comparing yourself with the men and women on magazine covers is hardly fair. Too many people who tell me they want to lose weight really want a body transformation! At birth, all of us were blessed with a certain body type or shape that, for the most part, can't be changed appreciably. Your body is one of these types:

Mesomorph: Muscular body with somewhat larger bone structure; generally the body shape is triangular (broad shoulders and narrower hips). Excess body fat is typically carried in the chest and back region.

Ectomorph: Slender body with narrow shoulders and hips (box-like shape), typically long legs, and no visible waistline. Excess body fat is carried in the waist region.

Endomorph: Round body shape, sometimes either an hourglass or pear-shaped figure. Excess body fat is carried in the hips or chest region.

Which body shape best describes you? Whichever it is, accept its shape and realize its potential. Staying in calorie balance will keep excess fat off your body frame. Regular exercise will keep your body toned and looking fit—no matter what your body type. But you can't expect to change your body from one type to another. Look at your body again—this is who you are, enjoy it. Do your best with what you have.

BODY FAT: HOW MUCH IS TOO MUCH?

Forget what the bathroom scale says—your weight doesn't matter. That's right ... it's not the number on the scale that matters. Your body fat percentage does matter. Overweight is a term you frequently hear describing a person's excess body fat. The term should really be "overfat." A person's body weight does not describe body composition adequately. A person might be "normal" in body weight based on height/weight tables but overfat based on body fat percentages. The distinction needs to be made, because being too fat increases the risk of heart disease, high blood pressure, diabetes, and certain types of cancer. But how much body fat is too much?

While the numbers span a broad range for what is a "normal" body fat percentage, most health authorities agree that for men 25 percent or more is obese, and for women the number is 35 percent. What is a normal or "ideal" body fat percentage? "Ideal" for what? First, both men and women must have a certain amount of fat for good health (for protection of organs and as an essential part of nerve cells and other tissue in the body). For men about 3 to 6 percent body fat is essential. For women the number is higher—about 10 to 13 percent. Women must maintain a higher percentage of body fat to support reproductive functions—menstruation and pregnancy.

With essential fat levels in mind, "normal" or "average" fat levels range from 11 to 18 percent for men and 18 to 25 percent for women. These average values correspond to a somewhat trim look with no obvious bulges around the waist. People who exercise regularly tend to have a lower percentage of body fat, particularly endurance athletes, who tend to have body fat percentages that read like shoe sizes. Carrying excess body fat can detract from performance. Running long distances, for example, is more difficult when carrying excess weight. Performance in other sports can be limited when an athlete has put on extra baggage beyond desirable levels. But a body fat level below the normal range doesn't necessarily mean better performance.

Body fat percentages for various sports are listed in Table 7-2. Compare these numbers to your own body fat number (see "What's Your Body Fat Percentage?" on page 218), but remember that each individual has an ideal body fat level for best performance.

Achieving a body fat level below what your body is designed for can leave you weak and susceptible to illness and injuries. Jim, a postal worker, came to see me about dropping his body fat level. He wanted to be leaner than his 14 percent body fat. As a serious cyclist, Jim felt he could improve his speed and endurance by dropping his body fat percentage. He had no difficulty in dropping his body fat to 10 percent through decreasing the percentage of fat in his diet and shaving calories here and there.

When Jim lost the weight to bring his body fat percentage to 10 percent, he began having problems with nagging aches and pains in his legs, which not only made walking his mail delivery route difficult, they decreased his cycling enjoyment. Jim's complaints—"I lost the spring in my step" and "Cycling is becoming a chore"—led me to believe his body fat change was not a positive one. Over a four-week period, he brought his body fat back to the original level, and his energy and performance returned. It was clear in Jim's situation that reduced body fat didn't mean better performance.

WHAT'S YOUR BODY FAT PERCENTAGE?

I suggest you get your body fat measured sometime soon. Having a ballpark figure will give you something to compare with average figures as well as a benchmark self-comparison over the years. If you are in the process of shaping up, slimming down, or just trying to maintain, you can use your body fat percentage as a way to monitor your health and performance.

Before you put yourself to the test, you should know the inside story on body fat testing. There is more than one way to measure body fat, and each method has its advantages.

Here's information on the latest body fat testing techniques available at health clubs and sports medicine facilities. Be familiar with the test you plan to use and ask the technician questions so you get the most information for your money.

Table 7-2 *TYPICAL BODY FAT FOR MEN AND WOMEN IN VARIOUS SPORTS*

Sport	Body Fat (%)	
	Men	Women
Cycling	6–14	12–22
Running	4–12	15–20
Swimming	5–10	14–25
Tennis	12–16	15–22
Triathlon	7–11	12–22
Weight lifting	6–16	10–18

Underwater weighing. This method measures the density of your body relative to the density of water. Fat floats, so the lighter you are in water, the more body fat you have. While this technique is considered very reliable, inaccuracies arise if the equipment is not well calibrated. In addition, if you are unable to exhale all the air from your lungs during the measurement, you become more buoyant and erroneously register more body fat. Note that underwater weighing was designed for adults (ages 20 to 50) and therefore is not as accurate for young children, adolescents, and the elderly.

Skinfold measurements. Skinfold calipers, resembling ice tongs, measure thickness of subcutaneous (under-the-skin) body fat. Skin is folded (pinched) at specific body sites—tricep, thigh, and subscapular (below the shoulder blade) skin folds. The thicknesses of all skin folds are converted into body fat percentages, using one equation designed for men and another for women. This method can be accurate if a skilled technician is taking the fold measurements.

Inaccurate results are commonly caused by rushed, sloppy measurements; also, you may have unusual body fat distribution, with more or less than normal fat stored at the traditional measuring sites. For instance, if your arms are disproportionately fat compared with other body sites, it might lead to overestimating of body fat. Yet the skinfold technique can be accurate for comparisons over time, provided you always have the same individual measure your body fat.

Bioelectrical impedance. This computerized method is new and can be done quickly, without getting wet or holding still for skinfold measurements. The body fat measurement comes from determining the resistance your body gives to an electrical current sent through body tissues from electrodes attached to your wrists and ankles. Water, found primarily in nonfat tissue, has little resistance to the electrical current. On the other hand, fat tissue provides greater resistance; thus, the more body fat you have, the more resistance to the electrical current.

This method of body fat determination is accurate, provided you haven't done anything to offset your normal water balance. You have abnormal water balance just after a long workout, after consumption of alcoholic beverages or coffee, or even after taking certain medications. Be aware that this method does seem to overestimate body fat for excessively overweight people, and this technique is not appropriate for the elderly.

Infrared interactance. This brand-new technique, originally used for meat grading by the U.S. Department of Agriculture, is based on the absorption of near-infrared light. A wand, connected to a computer, shines light directed to a specific site on the body. The computer calculates body fat by the way this light scatters and how much is absorbed. This method has been strongly criticized, since whole body fat is being calculated from information determined at just one site on the body. Because various individuals have somewhat different fat distributions, accuracy may be affected. While this method is quick (ten seconds), more information is needed from research to improve its acceptability.

Each method for determining body fat has its own specific advantages—comfort, convenience, accuracy. Choose one that feels right to you and have measurements taken at a reputable establishment. Resist comparing your body fat number with that of colleagues, since most methods have errors of two to five percent or more.

It is important that body fat measurements taken in subsequent years be compared with numbers obtained from the same fat-testing method. Above all, I suggest you keep in mind the body fat level at which you perform and feel your best. Remember, all science aside, how your pants fit is always a good indication of your body shape.

RUNNING ON EMPTY

Do you sometimes wish you could eat more than you do without putting on pounds? After all, you average about three or more exercise sessions a week and stay fairly active during the rest of the week. Still, you find yourself merely maintaining your weight, though you eat no more than your couch-potato friends.

If you think you deserve more food, you're not alone. From my experience, many active people of both sexes complain about having to eat less and exercise more just to maintain their weight. Studies confirm that high-mileage athletes can run on unusually low numbers of calories without losing weight. It's as if some athletes take on the efficiency of a high-mileage car, getting more miles to the calorie than before.

In theory, any activity such as sitting, walking, or running boosts calorie needs beyond basal levels. As shown earlier, the rate at which you burn calories during exercise depends upon your body weight, gender, and the intensity of your exercise. For example, if a man weighing 150 pounds was to run five miles each day at an eight-minute-per-mile pace, he would require an additional 500 calories per day to maintain his body weight. Unless he took in those extra calories daily, he should shed weight. While this may seem straightforward on paper, research shows the energy equation doesn't work for all athletes.

In one intriguing study, female marathon runners who averaged more than 65 miles per week consumed a mere 1,400 calories a day. Since normal-weight, sedentary women typically eat between 1,500 to 2,000 calories a day, it doesn't seem possible that the women runners could maintain weight and energy levels with so little food. Running 65 miles per week should have boosted calorie needs by approximately 800 calories a day.

Studies with different types of athletes show lower-than-expected calorie intakes. This calorie dilemma does seem to be more common in women athletes, but it tends to occur generally among those athletes who try to control their body weight: wrestlers, gymnasts, and dancers.

FINDING ANSWERS

Scientists search for reasons why some athletes can survive on so little energy. Some researchers feel that exercise may be just like a starvation of sorts and that the body responds by becoming more efficient with each calorie. Here are a few ways in which an active person may save some calories:

Basal metabolism slowdown. Regular exercise is commonly thought to increase basal energy expenditure. However, recent studies with energy-efficient athletes suggest that basal rates may not be increased. In fact, an athlete may burn fewer calories during sleep than a sedentary person does, suggesting a type of "hibernation" for athletes trying to conserve energy.

Weight loss. Cutting back on food may create an energy-efficient metabolism in both overweight and normal-weight people. Studies of obese individuals show that when they lose weight, their efficiency in drawing energy from the food they eat increases. They often require fewer calories per pound of body weight. Athletes who diet to control weight may simultaneously make their bodies more efficient at processing food.

Menstruation delays. Loss of regular menstrual function (amenorrhea) may be linked to low calorie intake. Several studies have shown that amenorrheic runners eat less than regularly menstruating runners with the same training mileage. While still unexplained, it may be that hormonal changes occurring in amenorrheic athletes improve metabolic efficiency and depress caloric needs.

Efficient digestion. Typically you absorb about 90 to 95 percent of a meal's energy, expending only a small amount of energy to process the food. People who overeat may absorb slightly less than efficient eaters do, since a few calories pass undigested through their systems. Overeaters may also expend more calories to process all that food. Underfed individuals, on the other hand, may process food more efficiently.

THE SOLUTION

If you face this issue of running on empty—eating fewer calories than you think you deserve—don't despair. You may be able to trick your metabolism to some extent by simply starting to eat slightly more over a period of weeks. I've had success with trying this on some athletes. Perhaps adding a few hundred calories a day, gradually, over a six-week span, will give your body time to adapt to the extra calories. Keep your eating pattern regular, too. Avoid skipping meals, because your body would treat that as a brief fast or starvation period, causing your metabolism to adjust to a possibly lower calorie-burning level in an effort to save energy.

HIGH-ENERGY WEIGHT LOSS

You have a good idea of where you stand—the weight at which you feel and perform your best. And if you know your body fat percentage, then you know whether shedding some pounds is in order. Vital to your top performance is feeling your best, and to feel your best you may have to drop some flab that is detracting from your performance potential. As you may already know, attempts at losing weight can leave you low on energy. But history shows that losing weight is a breeze compared with maintaining that weight loss. (Regaining the lost weight, and then some, seems inevitable.) But don't despair—Power Eating works!

Whether you are thinking of shedding 6 or 60 pounds, eating the Power Diet can get you there. The basic 60-15-25 diet is the ideal division of calories for weight loss as well as for top performance. Your switch to Power Eating shaves fat calories from your present eating style, and this alone may help in weight loss. Remember that extra fat calories in the diet are more "fattening" than extra carbohydrate calories.

Power Eating will also keep you feeling energized while you lose weight. With 60 percent of your calories coming from carbohydrate, your brain and muscles will be fueled for stamina. High-carb eating will keep you feeling your best, even though you're taking in fewer calories than you're burning. And despite everything you hear, burning more calories than you consume is the *only* way you can lose weight. Follow my tips for losing weight and keeping that weight off, and you will reach your best performance level and stay there!

TEN STEPS TO SUCCESSFUL WEIGHT LOSS

No matter how anxious you may be to slim down, your weight-loss program must follow these fundamentals if it is to succeed.
☐ Take in fewer calories than you're burning.
☐ Include regular exercise like walking or jogging.
☐ Incorporate changes in eating style, such as modifying the rate of eating or curtailing unplanned snacking.

Whether you go it alone or in a group with a weight-loss program, these ten steps will help you achieve your goal.

1. Get motivated. Whether it's 6 pounds or 60, don't attempt weight loss unless you're really ready to do what it takes. Motivation is the key to success.

2. Set a realistic weight-loss goal. Once you know your body fat percentage, or have figured out how many pounds you've put on since your thinner days, set a reasonable weight-loss goal that you can achieve safely. Deciding you have to lose 15 pounds in two weeks to fit into your bathing suit is not realistic, nor is it realistic to try losing an amount of weight that puts you below the normal body fat level at which you perform best. Set realistic goals so you can expect to succeed.

3. Cut no more than 500 to 1,000 calories daily. To lose a pound of fat, you must have a calorie deficit of 3,500. Cutting 500 calories a day should give you a weight loss of approximately one pound a week. This rate of weight loss is safe and will keep your energy levels up. The more calories you cut out, the more drained and listless you will feel. Losing two pounds per week (1,000 calories per day deficit) should be the maximum.

4. Track your eating style. Changing eating behavior is a challenge, and it doesn't happen overnight. Keeping a food diary to track your eating activities will help immensely. Write down not only what you ate but when, how you felt physically, your mood, how long it took for you to eat the meal or snack, whom you were with, and what you were doing (watching TV, reading, working, for example).

After a few days you will see a pattern in your eating style and be able to identify your danger times. For example, you may find that after work you snack on virtually anything you can find, because you are ravenous and usually upset about your workday. Your goal is to change this behavior by substituting different behavior, including a power snack in the midafternoon and a walk after work, to cut hunger and ease tension.

5. Exercise and exercise. Your goal is to burn more calories than you take in so that you will lose fat. Staying active and including regular exercise will do just that—burn calories. More than that, regular exercise helps you lose more fat and keep the muscle. You will feel better, more energetic.

6. Eat meals regularly. Skipping a meal to cut back on calories only leaves you feeling tired and hungry. You're more likely to overeat at the next meal, defeating your purpose of avoiding calories. Divide your calories among meals and snacks throughout the day, leaving your evening meal smaller than usual. Your breakfast should provide you with approximately one-third of your day's calories.

A typical case was a 40-year-old software specialist who wanted to drop about 10 pounds he had "collected" over the past year because his new job cut into his exercise time. I figured he needed 2,600 calories daily to cover his BMR and exercise needs. To lose one pound per week, he needed to take in 2,100 calories daily. This is how his calorie split for the day looked: breakfast (600), lunch (600), snack (300), dinner (600).

With this division of calories he didn't feel hungry in the morning, so he was able to resist his usual trip to the office vending machine. His afternoon snack also gave him a needed energy boost before his after-work workout.

7. Don't skip your favorite foods. Depriving yourself of those items that make eating worthwhile for you only results in a diet tougher to stick with. Include regular small portions of whatever your favorites are—cookies, candy, ice cream. If you have small amounts every so often, you're less likely to binge on these foods—bingeing makes you feel like a failure.

8. Set small goals for lifestyle changes. Allow yourself time to make changes in the way you eat and how you respond to food. It may take you weeks before you feel comfortable with your new eating plan. If you're not already exercising routinely, regular workouts may take some getting used to. Remember, you want permanent changes for lasting weight loss.

9. Keep track of your progress. Remind yourself of how wisely you ate or that you lost one pound last week. Note your feelings in a log or in your food diary so you can see the changes in your attitude toward yourself and toward others.

10. Reward yourself. Staying motivated during many long weeks of dieting is hard work. Giving yourself a treat every so often will keep your spirits up. But instead of an edible goodie, give yourself a reward that isn't food. Just about anything can be a reward as long as it's a treat to you: a new pair of workout socks or tights; a bubble bath; a trip to the movies; a massage— treat yourself to things that make you feel good, because after all, you're doing great!

WEIGHT-LOSS CLUBS

Despite our desire for speedy weight loss, most of us are aware, firsthand, of the commitment and effort it takes to lose weight and keep it off. And for many of us, getting help makes the job easier to tackle. This is why weight-loss programs and clinics have become so popular in recent years. Over $1.5 billion is spent annually on in-hospital clinics and other commercial programs.

Physician-supervised clinics like Optifast and group-effort programs like Weight Watchers offer many options to dieters—everything from liquid formulas and prepackaged meals to do-it-yourself menu plans. Many leading programs also educate dieters on how to keep weight off by applying lifestyle changes in exercise and eating habits. When choosing a program, look for one that fits your budget and personal needs. Prices range anywhere from about $8 a week with Weight Watchers to over $1,000 weekly for clinics with physician involvement and special products.

For long-lasting results, the best weight-loss programs include exercise and behavior modification classes to help dieters deal with real foods once off the supplement. Scientific studies show the key to sustained success is the incorporation of regular exercise that makes weight maintenance possible. Some people try these very-low-calorie diets on their own with over-the-counter products, such as Slim Fast. These diets are designed for use at 1,000 calories daily (diet product plus real food). However, unless you incorporate exercise along with techniques to change eating style, success on your own with this type of diet is not likely.

HOOKED ON LOSING

Have you been here before? I mean, have you lost weight only to regain it? Weight cycling, or yo-yo dieting, is all too common. It can be worse for your performance than if you were just to remain overweight. You're actually better off *not* losing the weight if you are unable to keep it off. Repeated bouts of losing and gaining weight have far-reaching effects on a dieter's health, metabolism, and longevity. And this troubling news is not reserved for just the big losers and gainers. Those of you battling with the same five to ten pounds year after year may also face specific health risks.

Studies with both people and laboratory animals suggest that each time weight is lost, this same weight is regained more quickly and efficiently—requiring fewer extra calories to gain back the same amount of weight. Also, subsequent attempts to take off weight regained become more difficult—requiring even larger sacrificial cuts in caloric intake to achieve the same weight loss as before.

Not only do yo-yo dieters regain quickly, they also change their body shape and composition—gaining back more fat. In the process, repeat dieters gradually increase their body fat and develop a stronger preference for fatty foods. Studies by Kelly Brownell, Ph.D., from the University of Pennsylvania Medical School, show that repeat dieters gain back more of the lost weight as fat instead of replacing the small amounts of muscle shed during dieting. Yo-yo dieters regain that extra fat around the abdomen, as opposed to the hip/buttocks region. This bulging midriff raises the risk for heart disease and high blood pressure.

Also, regainers report a greater desire for fatty foods, such as rich ice creams and fried foods, which boost weight gain and health problems. Additionally, large population studies find that men who repeatedly gain and lose weight are at greater risk of a heart attack than overweight men who haven't lost weight.

Regaining lost weight also happens to people who cut back on their exercise program or stop altogether. Work I did with Judith Stern, Sc.D., R.D., at the University of California at Davis, suggests that the body treats a hiatus from running the same way it treats rebounding from a crash diet. Large increases in fat metabolism occur after exercise is stopped for as little as three or four days. Evidence from animal studies suggests that ex-runners manufacture new fat cells while off their exercise routine. These new fat cells eventually fill with fat, making weight-loss attempts more difficult. Studies have shown that marathon runners and triathletes also experience rapid weight gain following just a one-week break in heavy training.

If you are on the weight-gain rebound, recent studies also suggest you're better off doing a little bit of activity while gaining rather than staying idle. Scientific studies show that while regaining weight, regularly exercising animals selected a diet lower in fat (25 percent of calories) compared with animals who didn't exercise while regaining (over 50 percent fat calories). These results may help explain why people previously very overweight will regain less weight when they maintain regular activity.

MAINTAIN INSTEAD OF REGAIN

The battle of the bulge is not over once the weight is lost. In fact, the toughest battle is yet to come—keeping lost weight off for good. You'll notice that most weight-loss programs will proclaim testimonials about clients who have dropped 20 pounds successfully, but you don't hear whether they were successful in keeping that weight off. Weight-maintenance statistics don't paint a rosy picture—over 90 percent of losers end up being gainers within a year of weight loss. Worse yet, they end up gaining more weight than they lost.

These statistics underscore the importance of making behavior changes that will help you modify your eating behavior and, ultimately, assist you in maintaining your new, healthier body weight forever! While it might take willpower to stay on a diet, it takes more than willpower to keep from regaining lost weight. Successful weight maintenance requires working toward new eating and exercise lifestyles, along with continued motivation to stay slim. Here are five key components to successful weight maintenance. Make them a part of your lifestyle!

1. Stay motivated. Remind yourself of the reasons you wanted to lose weight. Avoid getting into a trap of doing it for someone else's benefit—friend or spouse, for instance. Motivation has to come from within you, for your own personal reasons.

2. Keep active. Exercise and an active lifestyle are part of the daily routine for weight losers who manage to keep it off. Regular exercise has many benefits: It burns calories, keeps your body well toned, helps you cope with day-to-day stresses, and can lift you out of a bad mood by improving your sense of well-being.

3. Keep track of yourself. Just as you tracked your eating patterns before, keep track of them after weight loss. You may be tempted to go astray and sink back into your old habits again. Remind yourself what changes helped you lose weight and what bad habits contributed to your being overweight.

4. Stay involved. If you lost weight along with a friend or as part of a weight-loss group, then stay involved with those people. You can turn to them for support when you feel you are faltering.

Making exercise part of your daily routine is often easier when you make plans to exercise with someone regularly. Join a support group of weight maintainers to help you stay straight.

5. Adopt a reasonable and flexible plan. Weight maintenance must include a plan for daily eating and exercise. Knowing how many calories you need daily, for instance, will help you compensate for overeating at one meal by cutting back slightly at the next. Whether you track calories or food servings, work with a reasonable plan that allows you some flexibility, some leeway when you miss a few days.

LOSE WEIGHT WHILE YOU WORK

Your company may already have a worksite wellness program that can put you on the road to weight loss. More and more companies do this to promote healthful lifestyles. Not only can such a program save the company money in health-care costs and absenteeism but it can also improve employee work performance. Some companies even motivate employees with monetary rewards for weight loss. You can bring a weight-loss program to your worksite by contacting your personnel director and other employees to get something started. Here are a few organizations to contact for information on existing programs.

Weight Watchers at Work
Weight Watchers
79 Madison Avenue
New York, NY 10016
(212) 213-7084

LIFESTEPS
The National Dairy Council
Marketing Department
6300 N. River Road
Rosemont, IL 60018
(800) 426-8271

Johnson & Johnson Health Management, Inc.
1 Johnson & Johnson Plaza
New Brunswick, NJ 08933
(800) 443-3682

CHAPTER **8**

FINDING TIME TO EAT:
power-eating strategies

Demands on your time are incredible, forcing you to fit more and more into your schedule. But despite the hectic pace, you wouldn't have it any other way. Unfortunately, your ever-accelerating lifestyle makes it increasingly difficult to find time to eat properly. Your busy schedule requires stamina, but too often unforeseen situations interfere. Power Eating brings you strategies for success!

Whether you're on a plane, at a business lunch, or at home with only five minutes to get a meal, Power-Eating Strategies will work for you. They will put you in control and lead you to your top performance. Use my Power-Eating Strategies for dining out, fast-food eating, traveling (business and pleasure), breakfast meetings, and business lunches, plus round-the-clock home and work schedules.

I will show you how to put these strategies to work through easy-to-follow menus tailored to your busy schedule. Whatever your time demands, Power Eating will fit, giving you what it takes to stay ahead.

DINING-OUT TACTICS

Eating out has become a way of life—Americans average two out of every five meals away from home. Your eating options are endless, everything from pizza parlors, workplace cafeterias, and fast-food outlets to ethnic restaurants and elegant hotel dining rooms. Many people view dining out as a time to splurge, a time when nutrition doesn't count. But since eating away from home is now a regular part of your lifestyle, the food you get when dining out must do its part to fuel your performance; certainly it must not drain it. Use my basic dining-out tactics below, and you can easily eat for power at virtually any type of eating establishment.

Plan ahead. Collect menus from the places where you frequently dine. This gives you the opportunity to select a low-fat, energizing meal ahead of time so you can avoid what I call the feeding frenzy—a semi-delirious state brought on by a combination of hunger, fatigue, high-fat temptations, and mouth-watering aromas.

Plan on a balanced meal. If you order only a small salad or appetizer or only dessert, you may run short of power nutrients later. Balance your meal with small portions of a meat, fish, or vegetarian entrée, vegetable, salad, and bread, rice, or potato to get the boost you need.

Review the entire menu. Whether the menu is scribbled in chalk, printed on paper, or illuminated overhead, be sure to look over the entire selection. There may be a special "low-fat" section or a specialty that is low in fat and high in carbohydrates. Restaurants frequently feature healthful dishes on the menu and make an effort to add more choices to meet the demands of low-fat eaters.

Ask questions. Before you order, make sure you know what you are getting and how it is prepared. Many menu items that sound deliciously low in fat turn out to be low-performance high-fat disasters. For example, pasta dishes that come draped with cream sauces rich in performance-sapping fats are notorious for this. Become familiar with menu lingo that will help you zero in on hidden fats. (Check the "Menu Power Guide" below.)

Request changes or substitutions. Many restaurants welcome suggestions for menu changes and willingly prepare dishes in ways that will please you. For instance, ask for steamed veggies or fresh tomatoes along with your sandwich order instead of french fries, or request that your fish be grilled instead of sautéed.

Ask for sauces on the side. Often, most of the calories and fat in an entrée come from the rich sauce. Getting the sauce on the side will allow you to control the amount you eat. A request that the salad dressing be served on the side can easily shave 100 calories from a typical salad. Be cautious at salad bars—avoid creamy dressings and high-fat extras like bacon bits and grated cheese.

Ask for smaller portions. Restaurants tend to serve large portions of meat or fish, far more than the three ounces you need at a meal. Ask your waiter for a small serving of meat, with more salad, baked potato, or steamed vegetable as a trade-off.

Split an entrée with a friend. If you know a particular restaurant serves large portions, go there with a friend who will share the feast. Splitting a large entrée will leave room for salad and more carbohydrates such as bread or pasta.

Ask for low-fat condiments to spice up your meal. Some low-fat dishes may not have the kind of taste appeal creamy sauces and butter bring to virtually everything they are poured over. However, a dash of flavored vinegar, lemon juice, or a sweet, spicy specialty mustard can really liven up a dish of steamed vegetables or pasta.

Eat smaller portions if all else fails. If you enter an eatery that serves nothing but fatty hot dogs or similar nutritional minefields, you don't have to throw in your napkin! Simply eat smaller portions, and try to eat more fresh fruits and vegetables along with other quick carbohydrate foods, like whole-grain crackers, later in the day.

MENU POWER GUIDE

Making your way through a menu can be confusing, if not downright misleading. However, many restaurants now include information on calorie, fat, cholesterol, and sodium content of each dish as well as how the dish is prepared. Here is a simple refresher on common menu lingo so you can eat for power whenever you dine out.

The menu buzzwords that signal lower fat are: steamed, grilled, broiled, roasted, stir-fried, poached. The menu buzzwords that signal higher fat are: breaded, fried, creamed, au gratin, scalloped, hollandaise, Mornay, gravy, battered, sautéed, white sauce.

APPETIZERS

Best bets: Fresh fruit, raw vegetables and salsa dip, seafood cocktail (nonmayo sauce), vegetable-based soups—bean soups or minestrone (not cream type).

Avoid: Fried vegetables, chips, cream soups, pâté, cheeses.

SALADS

Best bets: Variety of greens, reduced-calorie dressings or lemon juice/flavored vinegar (request dressing on the side).

Avoid: High-fat add-ons such as cold cuts, cheeses, bacon bits, egg yolks, olives, creamy dressings.

MEATS/POULTRY/FISH

Best bets: Broiled, grilled, roasted, or poached (ask for meat "dry"—no butter or other added fat), unbreaded; ask for a lean cut of meat and trim away visible fat.

Avoid: Breaded, fried, or pan-sautéed meats, heavy sauces or gravy toppings, large portions (greater than four to six ounces).

PASTA/RICE/POTATOES

Best bets: Tomato sauces or other low-fat herb-seasoned toppings; boiled, baked, or steamed.

Avoid: Cream sauces or cheese toppings, egg noodles, fried, "home fried."

VEGETABLES

Best bets: Steamed, boiled, or stewed and served with lemon, herbs, or fancy mustards.

Avoid: Sautéed, fried, creamed, or added butter.

BREADS

Best bets: Plain French bread, dinner rolls, or other breads such as whole-grain or white, crackers, bread sticks, tortillas.
Avoid: Croissants, sweet rolls, fried breads.

DESSERTS

Best bets: Sorbets, fresh fruit, frozen yogurt, ice milk.
Avoid: Cheesecake, ice cream, pies, custards, pastries.

FAST-FOOD FEASTING

Eating breakfast, lunch, and dinner at fast-food outlets is not only commonplace—it's American! Every day, one in five Americans orders up a fast-food meal. But what are they ordering? Fat! Fast food is notorious for its fat content. In fact, the faster the food, the fattier it is likely to be. One McD.L.T., for example, contains more than 40 grams of fat, over half the suggested fat intake allotment for the day (see chapter 4). Fat makes the eater feel full and "satisfied"—precisely the goal of fast-food sellers.

Fast food is considered by most to be "junk food." Since we see little good nutrition in it, let alone performance-boosting carbohydrates, we tend to dismiss fast food as hopeless, so it doesn't seem to matter what we order. Take heart—fast food is part of our life, and you can make it part of your Power Diet.

You need a bit of savvy and some self-control to make this work. By making trade-offs between your all-time favorites and the lower-fat options, you can fit fast-food eating into your Power Eating routine. Here are some eating tips to help you get the fat out of fast foods.

BREAKFAST

□ Order pancakes with syrup (no butter) rather than egg/sausage sandwiches. You get more carbohydrates and save 160 calories.
□ Skip the sausage offered with egg sandwiches to save on fat calories. If you want meat with your egg, opt for the ham, which is much lower in fat than sausage or bacon.
□ Ask for *unbuttered* English muffins or toast.
□ Order orange or grapefruit juice with your meal.
□ Combine low-fat milk with fruit juice and an *unbuttered* English muffin for a speedy but complete breakfast.

Table 8-1 *SHAVE CALORIES AND FAT BY MAKING THE RIGHT FAST-FOOD CHOICES*

Instead of . . .	Order . . .	And Save . . .
Apple snack pie (McDonald's)	Soft ice cream cone (McDonald's)	65 calories, 9 grams of fat
Bacon and Cheese Potato (Carl's Jr.)	Broccoli and Cheese Potato (Carl's Jr.)	180 calories, 17 grams of fat
Beefy Tostada (Taco Bell)	Tostada (Taco Bell)	112 calories, 9 grams of fat
Burrito Supreme (Taco Bell)	Bean burrito (Taco Bell)	114 calories, 10 grams of fat
Coleslaw (Kentucky Fried Chicken)	Mashed potatoes (Kentucky Fried Chicken)	57 calories, 6 grams of fat
Combination pizza, 2 slices (Shakey's)	Cheese pizza, 2 slices (Shakey's)	174 calories, 4 grams of fat
Double burger (Wendy's)	Single burger (Wendy's)	210 calories, 14 grams of fat
Quarter Pounder with cheese (McDonald's)	Cheeseburger (McDonald's)	205 calories, 16 grams of fat

□ Take along extras like fresh fruit or dry cereal to boost your carbohydrate intake.

LUNCH/DINNER

□ When ordering burgers or fish sandwiches, tell them to hold the "secret sauce." Mayonnaise and tartar sauce, too, are loaded with fat.

□ Order an extra, plain hamburger bun (whole-grain, if available, for added nutrition) for additional carbohydrate.

□ Try vegetable-stuffed or chili-topped baked potatoes as an alternative to the traditional burger. Request that no melted margarine or butter be added.

□ Include a side order of salad with reduced-calorie dressing as part of your meal.

□ If you're having a salad bar meal, skip the high-fat toppings and extras like creamy dressings, bacon bits, olives, mayo-dressed potato and pasta salads, and sliced cold cuts.

□ Skip the french fries, or at least split an order with a friend.

□ Request that your tacos, tostadas, and burritos come without the sour cream.

□ Resist eating the fried tortilla shell that comes with the taco salad.

□ Drink low-fat milk instead of a milkshake to save on calories and fat.

□ Order a diet soda instead of regular soda to save about 150 calories per 12-ounce serving.

When you order at a fast-food outlet, choose the cheaper, "less fancy" item, since it's likely to be lower in fat and calories. For example, the standard hamburger at McDonald's has 257 calories and 11 grams of fat, while the Big Mac contains 562 calories and packs 35 grams of fat. Make it a rule to order the smaller item first; you always have the option of going back and ordering more. But if you add a crisp salad and a container of low-fat milk to the order, chances are you will feel fueled and ready to go.

ETHNIC EATING

Besides looking for convenience, you sometimes look for exotic tastes. Ethnic cuisines, such as Italian, Japanese, Chinese, Mexican, Thai, and Indian, are staples for many of today's on-the-go diners. But deciding whether a spicy Thai chili salad or Szechuan-style chicken dish is truly low-fat can be tricky, unless you know something about the cuisine. Virtually all ethnic cuisines have much to offer the Power Eater. It just takes knowing some basics about each cuisine's cooking style and ingredient staples.

As in "American" cooking (if there is such a thing), there are great high-performance picks along with not-so-healthful choices in every cuisine. The trick lies in not letting the multi-

Table 8-2 *WHAT'S HOT AND WHAT'S NOT IN ETHNIC FOODS*

Here is a guide to the right choices based on calories, fat, and cholesterol content.

Type of Food	Desirable	Less Desirable
Chinese	Wonton soup	Crispy duck
	Chinese greens	Egg rolls
	Steamed beef with pea pods	Chinese pork spareribs
	White or brown rice	*Kun pao* (fried chicken)
	Steamed fish	
Japanese	*Chiri nabe* (fish stew)	Tempura (fried shrimp or vegetables)
	Sukiyaki	
	Yosenabe (fish soup)	*Tonkatsu* (fried pork)
	Yakitori (grilled chicken)	*Age* tofu (fried tofu)
	Sushi, sashimi (raw fish)	
Thai	*Yum neua* (broiled beef with onions)	*Yum koon chaing* (sausage with peppers)
	Cold shrimp salad	
	Forest salad	Thai curries with coconut milk
	Po tak (seafood soup)	
	Larb (chicken salad with mint)	Deep-fried fish, duck, or chicken
Italian	*Cioppino* (seafood soup)	Cannelloni, ravioli
		Antipasto meats
	Pasta with marinara sauce	Fettucini Alfredo
		White clam sauce
	Pasta primavera (pasta with vegetables)	Garlic bread
	Minestrone soup (vegetarian)	

(continued)

Table 8-2—*Continued*

Type of Food	Desirable	Less Desirable
Mexican	Beans and rice	Fried chips, nachos
	Gazpacho	*Flautas*
	Steamed tortillas	Guacamole topping
	Black bean/vegetable soup	Beef, cheese enchiladas
	Plain tostadas and burritos	*Chilies relleños*
Indian	*Daal* (lentils)	*Bhatura* (fried bread)
	Karhi (chickpea soup)	*Ghee* (clarified butter)
	Chapati (tortilla-like bread)	*Korma* (rich meat dish)
	Khur (milk/rice dessert)	*Samosa* (meat and vegetables fried in dough)

syllabic menu lead you into error. As ethnic restaurants gain in popularity and consumer demand for tasty, healthful foods increases, menus tend to describe the contents of each dish. Also, most chefs are happy to modify almost any dish to suit your tastes and health needs.

For instance, to keep sodium intake down, ask for less soy sauce in a stir-fry dish; ask to have the Indian curry sauce served on the side to help keep fat in check; or substitute chopped tomatoes for sour cream on a tostada for added nutrition. Whatever your choice, feel confident about asking what's in a dish and how it's prepared. And don't be shy about requesting healthful additions, substitutions, and deletions.

TIPS FOR EATING ON THE ROAD

I've learned from my hectic travel schedule that a business trip can be more exhausting than a triathlon. But I've also learned how to cope with the stresses of travel and stay energized for days while working on the road. With my Travel Fitness tips and Power-Eating Plan for traveling, you can get the most out of your business trips and feel great whether you're gone for one day or one month.

STAYING FIT EN ROUTE

Part of the fatigue most people feel while traveling is due to the departure from their routine daily activity. Sitting on an airplane for hours or waiting in line at airports can leave you feeling exhausted even though you've done nothing strenuous. Day-long meetings and overnight stays at hotels also drain your energy levels. Here are some tips for staying fit on the road.

☐ Before you leave on your trip, plan on exercise. Call ahead to your hotel and ask about in-house facilities or local gyms. Then check your work schedule and block out exercise time.

☐ When you cross time zones in your travel, try to get on the new time schedule early. Set your watch to the new time a few days before you leave and start getting up in the morning at the "new" time. Then exercise and get to bed at your "new" time.

☐ Take along a pair of walking shoes in your carry-on bag or briefcase for a walking break whenever the opportunity presents itself. If you have a long layover at the airport, walk the length of the terminals to refresh your legs. Walk during breaks at meetings, or plan to walk the long way to and from your hotel.

☐ If time permits, jog around the airport parking lots and take advantage of the showers available to travelers at airports.

☐ If you're traveling for pleasure, make sure to include daily exercise activities as part of your vacation—you want to arrive home feeling refreshed, not sluggish.

POWER-EATING PLAN FOR TRAVELERS

Regardless of whether you drive, fly, or take a train, you need an eating plan to stay energized. Use these ten ways to beat travel fatigue with Power Foods:

1. Eat three square meals. Avoid skipping meals, particularly on the days you are en route, to keep energy levels up.

2. If you plan to fly, call ahead and ask to be served a low-fat meal. Most airlines offer low-fat, high-carbohydrate options. (Note: 24-hour notice is usually required for a special meal.)

3. Pack some Power Snacks in your carry-on bag—fruit, canned vegetable juice, bagels, low-fat crackers, fig bars or other low-fat cookies. These snacks make great alternatives to snack offerings on planes, or you can use them as meal add-ons to boost your carbohydrate intake.

4. Take along a plastic bike bottle filled with water. Plane travel can be extremely dehydrating due to the dry air that circulates during the flight. Frequent sips of water work against dehydration and the consequent headaches. Always accept fluids offered while in flight—your thirst level is not always an accurate indicator of your body's need for liquid.

5. Avoid alcoholic drinks and beverages that contain caffeine in flight, because these act as a diuretic—increasing fluid loss by promoting urine production. Just skipping alcoholic beverages while traveling may also help you adapt to new time zones more easily.

6. When you catch a meal or snack at the airport, choose high-carbohydrate foods in moderate portions to avoid feeling full, especially if you're due to continue flying and sitting for hours. Before you order at a snack bar or cafeteria, check the entire menu and apply the same dining-out tactics outlined earlier in the chapter. Many airports now offer alternatives to high-fat hot dogs and ice cream. Real fruit shakes and soft pretzels, for example, are great high-carbohydrate snacks that will keep you feeling energized during your travels.

7. At your hotel, ask to see the dining room's menu so you know what to expect if you eat there—or if you need to go elsewhere for healthful eating.

8. When you plan to travel into a different time zone, start to eat on the new time schedule while still at home to help your body become adjusted to the coming change.

9. Along with using the tactics given for eating at restaurants in "Menu Power Guide" earlier in this chapter, plan to eat slightly less than usual, since you probably won't be physically active as you travel. All that sitting and eating leads to weight gain and a bloated feeling.

10. Dining out can lose its appeal on long trips. Stop at a convenience store to pick up breakfast cereal, fruit, milk, and bagels and have a quick meal or snack in your hotel room for a change.

WORKDAY LUNCHING PLAN

Your midday meal fuels your afternoon on the job, and it can power you through an after-work workout. However, deadlines, meetings, and general mayhem at work or home often put you in such a time crunch that you're forced to grab a bite on the run—far short of what you need to meet the day's remaining challenges. Whether you lunch at your desk, dine out with co-workers, or choke down a meal over a business meeting, you can eat for success. Try this six-step plan to turn your lunch into a Power Meal.

1. Decide early on what you will be doing for lunch—a meal out with co-workers, a brown-bag lunch, a snack from the office vending machines, or a catered business lunch. If you know what's in store, you're more apt to choose foods for performance and finish your workday feeling great.

2. Never skip breakfast in anticipation of a big lunch. When you miss your morning meal, you feel ravenous by midday and you tend to stuff yourself. High-calorie lunches can make you sleepy and spoil your work performance in the afternoon.

3. When you go out for lunch, use the Menu Power Guide. Fast-food outlets and ethnic restaurants are popular lunch stops—check "Fast-Food Feasting" and "Ethnic Eating" earlier in the chapter for best picks.

4. Bring your lunch from home a few times each week. Lots of office workers are doing it these days. It's the perfect way to control what you eat and when. Pack a sandwich, fresh fruit, low-fat cookies like fig bars, and something to drink—flavored mineral water, for instance—for a power-packed meal. If you have access to a microwave oven at work (more than 70 percent of American workers do), use it to heat leftovers from home—pasta, a casserole, soup, or ready-made microwavable meals available at the grocery store.

5. When time is short, a well-chosen vending machine lunch can keep you going. Select foods that are low in fat—fresh fruit, low-fat yogurt, and whole-grain crackers, for instance. Many vending machines offer ready-made sandwiches and allow *you* to add the spread. If the choices seem limited at your workplace, ask for expanded vending machine offerings. Do your best to resist a

candy-bar-and-soda fix that leaves you low on energy later in the day.

6. When you lunch during a meeting, eat lightly. Too much food can make you feel sluggish and sleepy. Eat a midmorning snack to keep energy levels up if you know your business luncheon will involve more talking than eating.

FUELING STRATEGIES FOR MEETING HECTIC SCHEDULES

Everyone's day has the same 24 hours, but I'll bet you could use an extra few hours to squeeze in the errands you never seem to accomplish, finish up some loose ends at work, spend some time with your family, or just relax! Like me, you probably realize that there isn't enough time to do everything, but you give it a try anyway. With such a wild pace, day-long stamina is crucial to your success. You can have all the stamina you need through Power Eating. In fact, it works best for demanding schedules.

Since your day is anything but calm, you don't always find time to eat in a way that will fuel your endurance. Some days, for example, you may have to skip breakfast and dash out the door, settling for coffee at the office to keep going, only to fade fast as the morning drags on. I find that those who have little time to eat benefit most from Power Eating.

The two basic strategies that sum up Power Eating in the face of frenzied living are these: Routinely eat breakfast that fuels your performance, and use snacks to maintain energy levels during your day. By following my guide to Power Breakfasts and Fast-Track Snacking, you not only survive your hectic days but you finish each day with a sense of accomplishment and feeling of inner energy.

POWER BREAKFASTS

Breakfast can set the performance level for the rest of your day. I know your time is limited in the morning, and I know you may not have an appetite until your body gets going, but you need to fuel yourself after some 10 to 12 hours without food.

Those who skip breakfast are known to be less productive at work, to perform poorly on reading tests, and to show poor reaction time compared with regular breakfast eaters.

If you can spare just one minute from your morning routine, then you can command a Power Breakfast. Here are some tips on how to get your day off to a good start. (Remember that you don't have to eat breakfast at the kitchen table, nor do you have to eat the standard "breakfast" foods.)

Ease into the breakfast routine. If you rarely eat breakfast, don't try to change overnight. Start by eating a light breakfast once or twice during your work week and see how you feel. You'll notice that when you do eat breakfast, you're in control of your appetite when lunchtime rolls around instead of pouncing on anything edible, particularly high-fat, low-performance foods.

Keep quick-fix breakfast foods on hand. Stock a bag of bagels and a bag of English muffins (in the freezer so they don't get stale), plus fruit juice, fresh fruit or dried fruit, and some low-fat or nonfat milk. You're more likely to have something in the morning if you can get at it in a hurry.

Eat while you get ready. As you gather your things together for work, put on your makeup, or prepare the kids' lunches, you could be sipping on a power breakfast drink (½ cup low-fat vanilla yogurt blended with one banana, ½ cup orange juice, ½ cup strawberries, and a few ice cubes). Blender drinks like this are quick and easy and they provide you with lots of energizing carbohydrates plus protein, vitamins, and minerals.

Take breakfast with you. If for some reason you can't eat before you leave for the day, take something with you—a bagel breakfast sandwich made of lean ham and low-fat cheese along with a piece of fruit, for example. You can eat your breakfast while you poke along in the morning traffic, or bring it to the job. When you brown-bag breakfast from home, you're less likely to have a run-in with doughnuts, pastries, or other goodies that are regulars in many workplaces.

Keep breakfast foods at work. Many business places have refrigerators where you can stash small cartons of low-fat milk or fruit juice. These, with a stowaway box of cold cereal, are the makings of a great breakfast. Ready-to-eat breakfast cereals offer plenty of nutrition—fiber, vitamins, minerals—along with plenty of performance carbohydrates. In fact, studies show that people who regularly eat cereal for breakfast have a better overall vitamin and mineral intake than people who eat other foods for breakfast or skip breakfast altogether.

FAST-TRACK SNACKING

Besides starting your day with a power breakfast, look to snacking as a key strategy for keeping your energy level up and your performance on top. As schedules become tighter with responsibilities and obligations, square meals go out and snacks come in. Eight out of every ten people snack—snack foods constitute a $10 billion industry. By the end of this decade researchers say that most of us will get over half of our daily calories from snack foods. It's all due to the nationwide craving for convenience. And if you're like most snackers, you catch mini-meals throughout the day—after a workout, on the job in the afternoon, or in the early evening before you dash to a meeting.

Besides saving time, snacking can actually be good for you. Recent studies show snackers perform better in mental tests and have a lower risk for heart disease.

A Tufts University study suggests a midafternoon snack improves memory skills. Psychologist Robin Kanarek, Ph.D., tested college students on memorizing, math problem solving, reading comprehension, and alertness skills in the midafternoon, approximately 3½ hours following lunch. Fifteen minutes prior to testing, the students either ate a 200- to 300-calorie snack or had nothing at all.

The snackers and nonsnackers performed equally well on math and reading skills. But the memory and alertness skills of the snackers averaged 15 to 20 percent better than the nonsnackers. Kanarek suggests the high-carbohydrate snack may boost the energy supply to the brain, improving certain aspects of brain function.

Regular snacking may provide long-term health benefits, too. Large population studies suggest that people who "gorge" (eat one or two meals daily) may be at increased risk for heart disease.

(continued on page 248)

Table 8-3 *SELECT A SUPERIOR BREAKFAST CEREAL*

When choosing a breakfast cereal, read the label for fiber content along with vitamin/mineral fortification. Three to four grams of fiber per serving is suggested, and if your favorite cereal falls short of this amount, add a tablespoon of wheat bran or rolled oats for added fiber. Also, check the label for sugar content. Some cereals are more than half sugar. (Convert the cereal label lingo by using four grams sugar as being equal to one teaspoon.) Cereals that have a modest amount of sugar added—say one to three teaspoons—contribute less than 10 percent of your daily sugar intake. This table shows how your favorite cereal stacks up in terms of fiber, carbohydrates, sugar, vitamins and minerals. Serving size is 1 cup (approximately 1 ounce), except where noted.

Cereal	Calories	Fiber (g)	Carbohydrates (g)	Added Sugar	Vitamins and Minerals (%USRDA)*
Cold Cereals					
All Bran (⅓ cup)	70	10	22	1 tsp.	10–25
Bran Flakes	135	7.5	35	1 tsp.	10–45
Cap'n Crunch	160	0	32	4–5 tsp. or more	10–30
Cheerios	88	1.6	32	trace	10–45
Common Sense Oat Bran†	150	4.5	31	1 tsp.	15–40
Corn Flakes	100	1.0	24	1 tsp.	10–50

(continued)

Table 8-3—*Continued*

Cereal	Calories	Fiber (g)	Carbohydrates (g)	Added Sugar	Vitamins and Minerals (%USRDA)*
Cold Cereals					
Cracklin' Oat Bran†	150	10.0	40	2–3 tsp.	20–50
Fiber One (½ cup)	60	13.0	23	0	20–50
Frosted Flakes	147	0.0	35	4–5 tsp. or more	15–35
Grape Nuts (¼ cup)	110	2.0	23	0	10–25
Just Right Fiber Nuggets	150	3.0	35	1 tsp.	100
Mueslix-Bran	260	12.0	64	1 tsp.	6–40
Mueslix Crispy Blend	240	5.0	49	1 tsp.	10–25
NutriGrain Biscuits	135	6.0	35	0	10–25 (no added iron)
NutriGrain Wheat	150	4.5	36	0	10–25 (no added iron)
Product 19	100	1.0	24	1 tsp.	100
Quaker Oat Squares†	200	4.0	42	1 tsp.	20–60
Quaker 100% Natural‡ (¼ cup)	120	8.0	19	4–5 tsp. or more	4–10 10–35

Special K	110	0	20	1 tsp.	
Spoon-Size Shredded Wheat	135	4.5	35	0	4–10
Total	110	3	23	1 tsp.	100
Wheat Chex	150	3	35	1 tsp.	25–45
Hot Cereals					
Cream of Wheat	80	0.8	18	0	iron only—36
Kashi†	265	7.5	57	0	none
Oat Bran†	90	4.1	17	0	none
Oatmeal, instant Fruit 'n' Cream (1 packet)†	130	1.9	26	2–3 tsp.	15–25
Quaker Extra (1 packet)	100	2.4	17	0	100
Oatmeal, regular†	150	4.5	27	0	none
Total (1 packet)	90	2.0	18	0	100

NOTE: Data derived from product labels.

*Numbers represent the range for various vitamins/minerals found in each cereal.
†A good source of soluble fiber.
‡Added fat.

On the other hand, frequent snacking or "nibbling" is shown to lower blood cholesterol levels and, in some cases, leads to weight loss when compared to gorging.

The University of Toronto Medical School tested a typical three-meal-a-day eating routine against a snacking diet, measuring blood cholesterol and body weight changes. A group of 40-year-old men were fed identical amounts of food, either as 3 daily meals or 17 daily snacks (nibbling). Following two weeks of this eating pattern, no changes were noted in the men's body weights. However, an 8 percent drop in total blood cholesterol was observed in the snackers. More important, artery-clogging LDL cholesterol dropped almost 14 percent with the snacking routine, favorably lowering the men's risk for heart disease.

Beyond brain power and better heart health, snacking can energize your workout. Studies involving experienced cyclists show a 10 percent increase in endurance when a carbohydrate snack is eaten one hour before riding. Obviously, if hours have passed since you last ate, your body could use an extra shot of carbohydrate. Bread or fruit, for instance, will fuel your muscles and keep blood sugar levels steady to ward off fatigue.

Lunch at noon followed by a workout or perhaps a business meeting at 6:00 P.M., without allowing for a midafternoon snack, can leave you feeling weak and poorly motivated for a productive session. Time a high-carb snack for about two hours before exercising. This well-timed snack will kick in during your workout, stabilizing blood sugar levels and providing energy to exercising muscles and a hard-working brain.

Snacking provides the bulk of daily calories, carbohydrates, and other power nutrients for many people. But look at the snack-food aisle in your grocery store and what do you find? Fat, sugar, and salt. Most ready-to-eat snack foods are notorious for giving you lots of what you don't need and little in the way of vitamins, minerals, and power-boosting carbohydrates. Despite the lack of nutritional value, people gobble down over $5 billion worth of potato chips and tortilla chips annually and stash away candy, cookies, and salted snacks in their desks for daily coffee breaks. A recent survey, for instance, reported that over 50 percent of office professionals snacked on cookies and candy at break time.

Crackers and chips top the list of favorite packaged snacks. Typically, these foods don't bear a nutrition label, leaving consumers to guess from the finely printed ingredients list whether they are fat disasters. Even though some leading snack-food manufacturers have stopped using saturated fats like palm and coconut oil, many snack products still remain high in fat. Over 50 percent of the calories in a handful of chips are from fat, while most snack crackers pack at least 40 percent fat calories.

Other favorite snack foods—candy, cookies, ice cream, and salted snacks such as peanuts—contribute little to vitamin, mineral, or fiber needs. However, these foods do pack a wallop in calories that may leave you too full for a balanced meal later in the day. Besides calories and fat concerns, many ready-to-eat snack foods contain a hefty dose of sodium. For example, a one-ounce serving of pretzels, even though low in fat, has over 400 milligrams of sodium—one-fourth of your suggested daily intake.

But don't despair. You can bypass many of these snacking obstacles with a little snacking sense. Choose nibbles according to how they fit into your overall daily balance of fruits, vegetables, grains, dairy products, and meats. Eating a candy bar, for example, to perk up your afternoon supplies you with 200 to 300 empty calories (10 percent of your allotted daily total). Snacking on whole-grain crackers and vegetable juice instead gives you a dose of fiber, vitamins, and minerals, all vital for your performance.

Here are some tips to keep your snacking and performance on track:

Eat before you get too hungry. Waiting until you're ravenous leads to overeating—ten cookies instead of two! Control snack attacks and keep energy levels up by eating every few hours.

Keep nutritious snack foods on hand at work and at home. Stow away whole-grain crackers, vegetable and fruit juices, unsalted nuts, dried fruit, or unbuttered popcorn as quick snacks to ward off candy bar and cookie attacks.

Choose snacks with staying power if you're trying to hold out until the next meal. For instance, if you're grabbing a bite after a workout and your next meal is hours away, pick up skim milk and a muffin; a carton of yogurt and a bagel; or have whole-grain crackers and low-fat cheese. Such snacks not only hold you over for a few hours but they also help you bounce back from a workout.

Choose low-calorie items when nibbling before meals or in the evening. Stick with nonfilling fresh vegetables or fruits for nutritious before-meal snacks that won't spoil your appetite. Try vegetables dipped in low-cal dressing; air-popped popcorn; bread sticks; or a small piece of fruit as calorie-saving goodies for prime-time snacking.

Table 8-4 *SMART SNACKS*

Instead of . . .	Choose . . .	And Save . . .
2 cups regular microwave butter-flavored popcorn	2 cups air-popped popcorn	82 calories, 7 grams of fat
1 oz. potato chips	1 oz. low-salt pretzels	40 calories, 9 grams of fat (and get 50% more carbs)
1 cup premium ice cream	1 cup frozen nonfat yogurt	350 calories, 30 grams of fat
2 chocolate chip cookies	2 fig bars	30 calories, 5 grams of fat
4 high-fat crackers (Ritz) and 1 oz. whole-milk cheese	½ large square RyKrisp and 1 oz. low-fat cheese	90 calories, 10 grams of fat
2.25 oz. chocolate bar	2.25 oz. Power Bar	106 calories, 19 grams of fat
1 doughnut	1 bagel	145 calories, 17 grams of fat

SOURCE: Adapted from J. A. T. Pennington, *Bowes and Church's Food Values of Portions Commonly Used,* 15th ed. (Philadelphia: J. B. Lippincott, 1989).

NOTE: Some data derived from product labels.

Purchase single servings of packaged snack foods to control portion sizes. Eating right out of a large package of chips or pretzels may lead to nonstop snacking. (No matter what they say, people don't buy large-size bags just to save money.)

Choose low-fat, unsalted packaged snacks. Check the grocery store health-food aisle for high-fiber, low-fat, and low-salt versions of granola bars, pretzels, and chips. Look for the new lower-fat brand-name products, such as reduced-fat tortilla chips and "light" microwave popcorns, as healthful alternatives. Check Table 8-4 for snacking ideas that can save you fat and boost your performance.

CHAPTER 9

TAILORING YOUR POWER-EATING PLAN:
high-performance menus

Now it's time to put Power-Eating Strategies to work. The selection of quick and easy full-day menus that follows shows you how to do it in different situations—at home, at work, while traveling, or when getting ready for a 10-K run or bike ride.

Each daily menu lists the total number of calories along with the distribution of calories coming from protein, carbohydrate, and fat. Menus vary in calorie content to give you a variety of examples. Simply adjust meal portion sizes to meet your calorie needs. All meals are designed to pack plenty of carbs and key essential vitamins and minerals. You'll see that fast foods, restaurant meals, and vending machine goodies all fit into the Power Diet of 60-15-25.

POWER EATING AT HOME AND ON THE JOB

As I emphasized in the last chapter, demanding work schedules call for a sound breakfast and consistent eating throughout the day. The menus and the added breakfast suggestions that follow fill that need.

MENU 1

It's Tuesday morning, and your day is starting at a pace that is anything but calm. You have to be at work a half-hour earlier than usual to pull some things together before a luncheon meeting. You're planning on a brief gym workout after work, followed by a casual dinner with a co-worker at your place. Here's a Power Menu to keep your stamina at its peak all day long.

7:00 A.M.: Breakfast
1 toasted whole-wheat bagel spread with 2 ounces part-skim ricotta cheese
8-ounce glass of grapefruit juice

10:30 A.M.: Snack at Your Desk
6-ounce can V-8 juice with 2 bread sticks

12:30 P.M.: Luncheon Meeting
Grilled chicken breast salad (2 cups greens tossed with water chesnuts, celery, ½ cup Chinese noodles, and 3 ounces cooked chicken) with 2 tablespoons rice-vinegar dressing
1 large slice French bread
1 cup fresh fruit salad
Flavored mineral water

4:00 P.M.: Snack at Your Desk
1 banana and 1 RyKrisp cracker from vending machine

7:30 P.M.: Dinner at Home
Clam pasta: fresh marinara sauce (ready-made from supermarket) with added fresh herbs (basil and garlic) and canned chopped clams over 1½ cups cooked angel hair pasta with 1 tablespoon grated Parmesan cheese

1 cup microwaved broccoli with lemon and fresh tarragon

½ cup sliced cucumber and red cabbage salad tossed with balsamic vinegar and olive oil

1 cup reduced-fat frozen dairy dessert

ANALYSIS

Total calories: 2,300. Distribution: 65 percent carbohydrate, 18 percent protein, 17 percent fat.

MENU 2

Friday at the office, you're tying up loose ends before the weekend, so you plan to eat lunch at your desk. After work, you treat yourself to a night out at your favorite Chinese restaurant.

Breakfast

1 cup microwaved instant oatmeal topped with ½ cup sliced strawberries

1 cup 1 percent milk

1 toasted English muffin with 1 tablespoon apple butter

Lunch at Your Desk

1 microwave glazed chicken entrée

1 8-ounce carton low-fat milk

1 banana

2 fig bars

Afternoon Snack

2 ounces low-salt pretzels

12 ounces diet soda

Dinner at Chinese Restaurant

1 cup wonton soup with greens

1½ cups spicy beef with broccoli (3 ounces steamed beef)

1 cup steamed rice

1 cup stir-fry mixed vegetables (snow peas, mushrooms, bok choy)

2 fortune cookies

Plenty of Chinese tea

ANALYSIS

Total calories: 2,400. Distribution: 60 percent carbohydrate, 18 percent protein, 22 percent fat.

TEN POWER BREAKFAST SUGGESTIONS

To help start your day at a full run, here are some additional suggestions for carbohydrate-packed breakfasts that you can eat while getting ready in the morning, driving in the car, or on the job.

1. 390 calories, 61 percent carbohydrate
   2 NutriGrain frozen waffles spread with 1 tablespoon low-sugar jam
   1 cup skim milk
   1 peach

2. 475 calories, 77 percent carbohydrate
   8-ounce carton low-fat fruit-flavored yogurt
   1 whole-grain muffin (frozen type)
   8 ounces orange juice

3. 400 calories, 75 percent carbohydrate
   ½ cup raisin bran mixed with ½ cup muesli-type cereal
   1 cup 1 percent milk
   1 nectarine

4. 600 calories, 78 percent carbohydrate
   1 serving fast-food pancakes with 2 tablespoons syrup
   8 ounces orange juice

5. 380 calories, 66 percent carbohydrate
   1 toasted bagel spread with 1 teaspoon sweet mustard
   2 ounces turkey ham
   8 ounces pineapple-orange juice

6. 390 calories, 55 percent carbohydrate
   1 bran muffin (low-fat type)
   2 ounces part-skim mozzarella cheese
   1 banana

7. 400 calories, 52 percent carbohydrate
2 rice cakes spread with 2 tablespoons peanut butter
1 ounce raisins
1 sliced kiwifruit

8. 500 calories, 74 percent carbohydrate
Blender drink: 1 cup low-fat vanilla yogurt, ½ cup
    orange-pineapple juice, ½ cup sliced strawberries, 2
    ice cubes
2 slices cinnamon bread with 1 teaspoon margarine

9. 480 calories, 70 percent carbohydrate
Pita melt: 1 whole-wheat pita bread topped with 1 ounce
    mozzarella cheese
¼ cantaloupe
8 ounces cranberry juice

10. 400 calories, 60 percent carbohydrate
Scrambled-egg-and-muffin sandwich: 1 egg and two egg
    whites, 1 toasted English muffin, 1 teaspoon
    margarine
1 8-ounce can vegetable juice
1 peach

POWER EATING ON THE ROAD

Fueling your performance on the road is a challenge because your daily routine is ruined, with little resemblance to home. Look back to "Tips for Eating on the Road" on page 238 for advice on meeting the challenge. Sticking to your normal eating routine and choosing foods that fit into the Power Foods scheme will keep you feeling energized while you're on the road. Here are two full-day menus for traveling, along with some airport and on-the-road snack suggestions.

MENU 1

You're about to start a three-day road trip packed with late-night dinners, early-morning breakfast meetings, and day-long work sessions. The early-morning flight has you at the airport by 7:00 A.M.

Breakfast: While Waiting for Your Plane
1 bran muffin

1 cup orange juice
1 cup low-fat milk

Snack on Airplane
2 whole-grain crackers with 1 ounce cheese
1 cup tomato juice

Late Lunch after First Meeting
Deli sandwich: 2 ounces roasted turkey breast, 1
teaspoon mustard, tomato slices and greens, 1 sour
French roll
12-ounce can fruit juice and sparkling water
1 cup fresh fruit salad

Dinner at Restaurant with Client
Grilled tuna with fresh herbs
Steamed summer squash
1 cup rice pilaf
Small dinner salad with 1 tablespoon house vinaigrette
dressing
1 decaf café au lait made with ½ cup low-fat milk

ANALYSIS

Total calories: 1,800. Distribution: 60 percent carbohydrate,
16 percent protein, 24 percent fat.

MENU 2
While at your hotel you plan to do some work in the evening,
so you will use room service for dinner.

Breakfast in Hotel Dining Room
1½ cups oatmeal with ½ cup fresh seasonal fruit (sliced
strawberries or a peach), ½ cup low-fat milk, and 2
teaspoons brown sugar
2 slices toast spread with 2 tablespoons jam

Lunch: Business Meeting with Clients
2 cups pasta salad with 2 ounces grilled shrimp,
1 cup mixed steamed vegetables, and ¼ cup light
cheese sauce

2 pieces French bread
12 ounces herbal iced tea

Snack: Quick Bite While on Your Way to Another Meeting

1 large soft pretzel spread with 1 tablespoon mustard
12 ounces diet soda

Dinner in Your Hotel Room after a Long Day and a Quick Workout in the Hotel Exercise Room

1 small cheese pizza topped with peppers and onions (or your favorite veggie)
1 dinner salad with reduced-calorie dressing
12 ounces flavored mineral water
1 cup frozen yogurt with fresh fruit topping

ANALYSIS

Total calories: 2,400. Distribution: 64 percent carbohydrate, 16 percent protein, 20 percent fat.

HIGH-POWERED SNACKS FOR THE ROAD

The following snacks pack well in your briefcase or carry-on bag and are great performance boosters when you're racing against the clock. You can plan ahead and take these snacks with you, or stop at a vending machine, airport snack shop, or quick-stop food store while you're on the road.

□ Single-serve box ready-to-eat cereal
□ Small packages low-fat snack crackers
□ Bread sticks
□ Canned fruit juice
□ Dry-roasted nuts
□ Popcorn without butter
□ String cheese with crackers
□ Small box raisins
□ Fresh fruit: orange, apple
□ Small can vegetable juice
□ Small package low-fat cookies
□ Small package low-salt pretzels
□ Graham crackers
□ Small package dried fruit: apricots, prunes, and peaches

POWER MENUS
FOR WORKOUTS AND RACES

You know from your own experience that what you eat before a workout or race event, such as a 10-K run, affects your performance. In chapter 2, I outlined the principles of high-carbohydrate eating along with what's best to eat and to avoid before exercise. The key to top-notch performance is the proper timing and the right amount of carbohydrates eaten before and during exercise. Timing of carbohydrates after a workout is also key to your recovery and performance. The menus that follow put these Power Eating principles to work for you.

MENU 1

Your plans are to meet an old college friend back in your hometown and run in the annual 10-K. After leaving work early Friday afternoon, you drive a few hours and stay the night close to the race start. Here is what you should eat the night before the event, race-day morning, and following the run.

Dinner the Night Before: At a Local Pizza Place

> 3 slices cheese pizza
> 1 medium-size dinner salad with tomatoes and
>   cucumbers with 1 tablespoon reduced-calorie dressing
> Plenty of water
> Frozen yogurt in a cone

> *ANALYSIS*
> Total calories: 955; 62 percent carbohydrate.

Race-Day Morning: Eat Two to Three Hours before Race Start

> 2 toasted English muffins with 2 tablespoons reduced-
>   sugar jam
> 1 banana
> 8 to 12 ounces water

> *ANALYSIS*
> Total calories: 430; 83 percent carbohydrate.

After the Race: Eat within about One Hour after Finishing
    1 plain bagel
    8-ounce bottle fruit juice and sparkling water
    1 ounce dried fruit

ANALYSIS

Total calories: 310; 85 percent carbohydrate. (See "Recovery Eating: The Right Way to Recharge after Exercise or Hard Work" on page 68 for six steps to fast recovery after exercise.)

FURTHER SUGGESTIONS

Check "Prerace Menus" on page 67 for more prerace meal suggestions. Remember to avoid unusual foods when traveling to races so as not to risk stomach upset. Drink coffee or tea on race-day morning only if you are in the habit of doing so. Coffee and tea, along with high-fiber foods such as bran cereals, tend to precipitate intestinal discomfort during exercise. Because of this, you should modify what you eat on race day morning to minimize the number of bathroom stops along your run.

MENU 2

As part of your summer vacation, you are going to go on a 75-mile bike tour with a group from work. Preparing yourself for this event requires weekend bike rides and some carbo-loading on the days before the tour. Check Table 2-7 for more on carbo-loading how-to's. Also, what you eat during this long ride is crucial to your performance. Here's a high-carb menu for the day before the event, along with some snacks to take along in your fanny pack to keep energy levels up during your ride.

Breakfast
    2 cups whole-grain cereal with 1 cup 1 percent milk and ½ cup blueberries
    2 slices toasted cinnamon bread with 2 tablespoons apple butter

Lunch at a Fast-Food Outlet
    1 large baked potato topped with 1 cup steamed broccoli and ½ cup cheese sauce

1 hamburger roll
12 ounces orange juice

Snack
4 cups air-popped popcorn
12 ounces diet soda

Dinner
2 cups rice topped with 1 cup refried beans (vegetarian style), chopped fresh tomatoes, and cilantro plus 1 ounce grated low-fat Monterey Jack cheese
2 cups mixed green salad with 1 tablespoon low-calorie dressing
2 flour tortillas
1 cup fruit sorbet

ANALYSIS
Total calories: 2,600. Distribution: 74 percent carbohydrate, 14 percent protein, 12 percent fat.

SNACKS FOR THE RIDE

During a long bike ride, you need carbohydrate energy to power your leg muscles along with plenty of fluids to stay cool. Here are some suggestions for energizing foods that pack well for the trip.

□ Fig bars
□ Dried pears, apricots
□ Meal-on-the-Go snack bar
□ Ready-to-eat breakfast cereal (Corn Chex, Quaker Oat Squares)
□ Easy-to-pack fruit: bananas, grapes
□ Raisin-filled biscuits
□ Low-fat granola bars
□ Power Bar
□ Vanilla wafer cookies spread with low-sugar jam
□ Fruit roll-ups

CHAPTER **10**

A LITTLE PLANNING GOES A LONG WAY:
get ready for power eating

You now know the Power Diet basics and how to Power Eat in virtually any situation with just about any combination of foods. All of my guides, tips, and steps focus on putting the Power Diet to work for you—regardless of the challenges you face. You should be confident about your ability to optimize performance and increase stamina even when your day is packed with activity. Now get your home ready for Power Eating by following my simple planning tips:

□ Power Shop at the grocery store—know what to look for in each aisle and how to interpret food labels.

□ Select foods that are not only quick to fix but safe to eat.

□ Stock your kitchen with basic foods and cooking utensils essential for Power Eating.

□ Put your microwave to use as vital part of your Power Eating routine.

□ Select the ten Power Foods to keep on hand for performance eating anytime.

POWER SHOPPING

You can get just about anything—fresh-baked breads, prepared pastas, exotic produce, even oven-ready meat loaf—at any time of day or night at most supermarkets. If you're an average shopper, you spend about 20 percent of your income on groceries, shop at least twice a week, and take advantage of in-store delis and bakeries. But are you Power Shopping?

Do you go through the supermarket filling your cart with high-performance, quick-to-fix foods for the week? Not an easy task with the some 10,000 items fighting for your attention—some with confusing food labels, others with no labels at all. You may also have concern about which foods contain questionable additives and pesticides or present the risk of bacterial contamination.

If you use my Power Shopping strategies and tactics, you can make your way through supermarket aisles efficiently, choosing healthful, high-powered foods from every section—deli counter, bakery, or frozen foods.

MAP OUT YOUR SHOPPING TRIP

Don't just *do* it—strategize your grocery shopping if you really want to maximize the results of your efforts. Here's how:

□ Plan to shop after you've eaten, even if this means grabbing a quick snack before you hit the aisles. Shopping on an empty stomach can mean a grocery cart overflowing with high-impulse, low-nutrition goodies.

□ Make a list, or at least outline in your mind what you want to buy. That way you'll stay on track, finish your shopping sooner, and arrive home with groceries that fit into your Power Eating plan.

□ Read food labels and keep the "nine rule" in mind—every gram of fat packs nine calories. Simply multiply the grams of fat per serving by nine and compare this number to the total calories per serving. You're aiming for 30 percent or less fat calories in every product. Also remember that *a teaspoon of fat is equal to five grams.* Knowing this helps you to visualize how much fat is hidden in foods like cookies and snack crackers.

START FRESH

Your first stop should be the produce aisle, to load up on vitamin and carbohydrate-rich fruits and vegetables. Your goal is at least five daily servings of fruits and vegetables. If you fill your cart with tasty fruits and crunchy vegetables, you won't be tempted to load up on sweets and other goodies as you walk through the store.

Look for crisp, dark-green lettuces rich in beta carotene for salad makings, along with add-ons like tomatoes, bean sprouts, green onions, and radishes. Select at least three cruciferous veggies (broccoli, cabbage, brussels sprouts, bok choy).

As you pass through the produce section, pick up citrus fruits and berries, along with green peppers, tomatoes, and potatoes, to insure that you get your daily dose of vitamin C. Try different in-season fruits each week for variety and added nutrition. Buy a bag of potatoes for the week—they make a great microwave meal topped with steamed veggies and low-fat cheese. You can even refrigerate extra baked potatoes for quick high-carb snacks.

MAKE THE MEAT
AND FISH MARKETS PAY OFF

Over the past few years, meat and seafood counters have changed dramatically. Your options have broadened to various new cuts of lean meats, oven-ready marinated cuts of poultry, fish, and beef, as well as expert help from the person behind the counter on how best to prepare lower-fat meat cuts and various types of fish for better flavor. Here is how to shop these markets for Power Foods:

☐ Buy ready-to-cook poultry, fish, or beef that has been skinned or trimmed of visible fat. Avoid breaded or stuffed items that may contain added fats.

☐ Select skinless poultry (or skin it yourself before cooking). Try ground turkey or chicken as a low-fat substitute for ground beef. (Check the label to see if the poultry skin is included in the ground product, or ask at the counter.)

☐ Look for Select grade beef, which is lower in fat than Prime or

Choice cuts. Ask your butcher for "Total Trim" meat cuts, which have virtually all of the visible fat removed and are sold in smaller portions to help control serving sizes. Remember, a maximum of six ounces of meat daily is your goal.

☐ Virtually any fresh fish is a great buy. Salmon, mackerel, and other cold-water fish are higher in fat than most, but they provide fish oils (omega-3's) which help to lower blood cholesterol and blood pressure in some individuals.

DELI DELIGHTS

In-store delicatessens are booming. Grocery stores are looking more like restaurants these days, offering ready-made pasta salads, roasted chicken and ribs, and a host of other dishes that can be packed up in minutes to take out. Since these foods aren't labeled you need to use your own sound judgment, and not just your eyes, nose, and stomach, when you choose. Follow these tips and you're on the right track:

☐ Look for pasta salads that are light on oils and mayonnaise. Plan to add more veggies at home to help dilute any excess fats.

☐ When buying lunch meats, choose roasted chicken or turkey, lean ham, or roast beef. If you are watching your sodium, ask for a low-salt item.

☐ Ready-to-cook fresh pastas along with fresh sauces are a great deli choice. Ask what's in the sauce and avoid cream-base mixtures. At home, you can add fresh tomatoes and herbs to red sauces as a nutritional boost to your meal.

☐ Select fruit salads that look fresh rather than those drenched in syrup or creamy dressings.

☐ Grocery store salad bars make for a quick lunch or take-home meal, but beware of high-fat add-ons like croutons, bacon bits, cheeses, and fat-laden salad dressings.

DAIRY DELIGHTS

Use your label reading skills at the dairy case to select low-fat cheeses, yogurt, and milk. Dairy products supply you with most of your daily calcium and riboflavin needs along with quality protein. If you make a few substitutions and try some of the new reduced-fat dairy products, you can easily get dairy product goodness without the extra fat. Put these guidelines to work right away:

□ Select skim or 1 percent milk. Using the "nine rule" on low-fat (2 percent) or whole milk, you'll see that over 30 percent of the calories come from fat in these milk products.

□ Select a variety of low-fat or nonfat yogurts to keep on hand for breakfast (eat along with a bagel and a piece of fruit), lunch, or a quick snack. Use plain yogurt instead of sour cream in recipes. Those who can't drink milk (lactose intolerant) may find small amounts of yogurt agreeable; lactose-free dairy products are also available (but check the label for fat content).

□ Try part-skim ricotta cheese in place of cream cheese on your bagels or in recipes—it's lower in fat and a much better protein source than cream cheese, which is virtually all fat.

□ Cheeses are generally 60 percent fat calories or more. Select lower-fat cheeses like part-skim mozzarella or reduced-fat cheddar and Monterey Jack cheeses.

□ When buying margarines, look for those that have liquid vegetable oil as the first ingredient. This will help lower your saturated fat intake. Diet margarine, still 100 percent fat, contains water, which effectively reduces calories per teaspoon— make sure you still use small amounts as if it were regular margarine.

BAKERY GOODIES

If you're a cookie monster, an in-store bakery can create the irresistible urge to jump the counter and attack. If fresh bread is delivered to your local grocery store daily, try to calm your desires with fresh-baked whole-grain breads. And if you can exercise control, some goodies at the counter can be a Power Eater's friend. Here's what to do:

□ Select whole-grain muffins, breads, bagels, and rolls for added fiber and nutrition. Ask what's in unlabeled bakery items to get an idea of added fats.

□ If you're after sweets, select un-iced angel food cake, ginger snaps, or molasses cookies, which are generally lower in fat and cholesterol.

□ Try the line of fat-free bakery items (cakes, cookies, coffee cakes) from Entenmann's Bakery. These products are less than

100 calories per serving, and though they contain sugar, they are a carbo-lover's dream.

CANNED, BOXED, BOTTLED, AND BAGGED

Affectionately called dry groceries by supermarket personnel—cereals, canned foods, salad dressings, dry pasta, dry beans, and bottled juice drinks and sodas, to name a few—they make up about one-third of your weekly grocery bill. Before you reach for any of these items, simply read the ingredients list and look for fat calories (and sodium content, if you're keeping an eye on salt). Profit from these simple hints:

□ Breakfast cereals are a great anytime food, loaded with carbs, vitamins, minerals, and fiber. Choose cereals with at least three to five grams of dietary fiber and less than two grams of fat per serving. If you like high-sugar cereals, plan to mix your favorite with a low-sugar variety for more complex carbs.

□ Buy canned fruits that are water packed to avoid extra sugar, and select canned vegetables (reduced-salt versions) like kidney and garbanzo beans that can be added to salads, stews, casseroles, or soups.

□ Canned vegetarian chili, water-packed tuna, and refried beans are all good low-fat protein choices to keep stocked in your cupboards.

□ Choose reduced-calorie salad dressings or no-oil versions to save on fat. Read labels to compare which brands are lower in sodium.

□ Dry pastas and beans are a must for Power Eaters. Keep a package of each in your pantry for a high-carb meal. To save time, quick-cook the beans instead of soaking them overnight (read package directions). Packaged pasta salads can be fat disasters: Check the label for fat grams (1 teaspoon = five grams of fat = 45 calories).

□ Look for quick-cooking brown rice as another high-carbohydrate staple for your kitchen.

□ Most bottled fruit drinks are only 10 percent fruit juice. Select bottled or boxed fruit juices that are 100 percent fruit juice for superior vitamin and mineral content.

□ Look hard at the labels of packaged snack foods like crackers, cookies, popcorn, and potato chips. Typically these foods con-

Table 10-1 *FROZEN DINNER LINEUP*

When choosing a frozen dinner or entree, aim for 300 calories, with 30 percent or less fat calories (10 grams of fat or less) and less than 800 milligrams of sodium. With a few meal add-ons like a warmed whole-grain roll and a fresh green salad, you have a great Power Meal in minutes. Here's how the leading "light" frozen dinner and entree lines stack up on fat and sodium.

Dinner	Calories	Calories from Fat (%)	Sodium (mg)
Budget Gourmet Light	270–300	17–28	670–810
Budget Gourmet Slim Selects	260–290	17–47	560–1,130
Healthy Choice	210–310	4–20	260–560
LeMenu Lightstyle	220–280	14–29	600–830
Stouffer's Lean Cuisine	190–280	17–43	400–1,190
Stouffer's Right Course	240–320	20–29	550–590
Weight Watchers	180–370	7–55	350–1,100

NOTE: Data derived from product labels.

tain at least 40 percent fat calories, even though the label may claim "cholesterol free" or "contains no tropical oils."

FROZEN WONDERS

The frozen foods aisle offers a growing number of timesaving complete meals, snacks, desserts, and side dishes that can be microwaved in minutes. Read the labels carefully so you can make the best choices. Select frozen dinners that are 300 calories or fewer, contain less than 10 grams of fat, and have 800 to 1,000 milligrams or less of sodium. With the lines of Healthy Choice and Stouffer's Right Course you have many to choose from.

Check Table 10-1 for your favorite frozen dinner lines (or shelf-top variety) and see how they compare on fat calories and sodium.

If you are shopping for kid-style frozen dinners, apply the same standards you would in selecting one for yourself. Some dinners are over 40 percent fat calories, loaded with sodium, and short on the fiber, vitamins, and minerals your child needs for good health. Look over Table 10-2 for children's frozen dinner comparisons.

Choose fruit sorbets, fruit bars made with the real thing, and ice milk or reduced-fat ice creams for low-calorie/low-fat sweets. Most bakery-type desserts, such as cakes and pies, tend to be high in fat. Use the "nine rule" on frozen muffins and cakes to avoid hidden fats. Check Table 10-3 for low-fat cool treats.

For vitamin-packed meal add-ons, choose frozen vegetables like broccoli, green beans, and spinach. Avoid vegetables packed in cream or butter sauces.

You don't have to go it alone when you shop. Many major grocery store chains offer some type of shopping assistance. Safeway, for example, has a shelf labeling program to identify food items that are low in fat, cholesterol, and sodium. Better yet, you can get in-store guided tours like Supermarket Savvy, providing aisle-by-aisle advice on food selection to help you shop for better health.

USING FOOD LABELS FOR POWER EATING

When you shop for groceries, use food labels to find out which products fit into the Power Diet 60-15-25 scheme. You're after

Table 10-2 *KIDS' MICROWAVE MEALS*

Representative dinners from three major lines show what's available. Watch out for high fat and sodium levels.

Dinner	Calories	Fat (g)	Calories from Fat (%)	Sodium (mg)
Banquet Kid Cuisine				
Cheese Pizza	240	4	15	390
Fried chicken	430	23	48	660
Macaroni and Cheese with Franks	380	14	33	1,000
My Own Meals				
Chicken, Please	220	4	16	550
My Favorite Pasta	230	8	31	480
My Meatballs and Shells	210	9	39	440
Tyson Looney Tunes Meals				
Daffy Duck Spaghetti and Meatballs	320	10	28	650
Wile E. Coyote Hamburger Pizza	320	11	31	660
Yosemite Sam BBQ Chicken	280	12	39	510

NOTE: Data derived from product labels.

foods low in fat (less than 30 percent fat calories) and high in carbohydrate. You also want to keep saturated fat, sodium, and cholesterol intake in check, and make sure you're getting the recommended 25 grams of dietary fiber daily. Food labels list all that information. The Food and Drug Administration (FDA) food labeling regulations of 1990 made labels less confusing and more responsive to the health-seeking consumer's needs.

You can use food labels to help you identify the foods that fit into your Power Eating style. Here's what to look for on packaged foods, and tips to help you decide whether a specific food meets your needs.

Calories. The number of calories per serving is listed at the top of the food label. Compare this number with your allotted calories for the day. This way you can identify a food that packs a lot of calories, and compare the calories to the quantity of nutrients this food supplies. Also, look at the serving size. Some products list a serving size much smaller than you are used to.

Protein. The amount of protein in a food is listed in grams. (Check chapter 3 for how many grams of protein you need for top performance.) Surprisingly, many frozen dinners fall short on protein, providing less than 15 grams per dinner (about one-quarter to one-fifth of an average protein requirement).

Carbohydrate. You're after a diet high in carbs, so use the number listed when adding up the grams of carbohydrate you've eaten in a day. The number of carbohydrate grams is particularly helpful when comparing carbohydrate-rich foods, such as pasta dishes and other grain products. But don't forget that sugar content is shown as carbohydrate.

Fat. Perhaps the most important bit of information on a packaged food is the number of fat grams contained in it. It's often difficult to determine if a food is high in fat by looking at it or even by tasting it. If you know the amount of fat per serving, you can calculate the percentage of fat calories by applying the "nine rule" described earlier in this chapter.

Some food manufacturers voluntarily list fat calories. Soon the FDA will make this mandatory so consumers can determine if specific foods are high in fat. Saturated fat is also listed on some food labels, identifying those that should be avoided or used in moderation. *(continued on page 274)*

Table 10-3 *IS IT COOL?*

See how your favorite frozen treat stacks up in terms of calories from carbs and fat.

Product	Portion	Total Calories	Calories from Carbohydrate (%)	Calories from Fat (%)
Crystal Light reduced-calorie bar	1.8 fl. oz.	14	57	0
Dole fruit and juice bar	2.5 fl. oz.	70	97	0
Dole sorbet	4 fl. oz.	110	100	0
Froz Fruit fruit bar	4 fl. oz.	70	91	0
Jell-O Gelatin Pops	1.8 fl. oz.	35	91	0
Simple Pleasures nonfat dairy dessert (Simplesse)	4 fl. oz.	140	71	0
Weight Watchers reduced-calorie bar	2.75 fl. oz.	100	72	9
Knudsen yogurt pops	3 fl. oz.	90	84	10
Dreyer's frozen yogurt	3 fl. oz.	80	75	11
Dole Fresh Lites Bar (sugar free)	1.65 fl. oz.	60	67	15

Rhapsody Farms frozen yogurt	½ cup	89	67	20
Yoplait frozen yogurt	3 fl. oz.	90	71	20
Jell-O Pudding Pops	1.75 fl. oz.	80	55	22
Ice milk	½ cup	100	60	27
Jell-O Fruit and Cream Bars	1.8 fl. oz.	60	50	30
Breyers Light ice cream	4 fl. oz.	110	51	32
Rice Dream, nondairy dessert	½ cup	140	60	32
Ben & Jerry's light ice milk	4 fl. oz.	240	50	38
Sorbet and cream	4 fl. oz.	200	54	41
Ice cream, regular	½ cup	135	47	47
Häagen-Dazs ice cream	4 fl. oz.	290	40	53
Tofutti nondairy dessert	½ cup	210	38	56

NOTE: Data derived from product labels.

Cholesterol. In an effort to help consumers stay within the suggested maximum intake of 300 milligrams of cholesterol daily, some packaged food products list the cholesterol content on the label. The FDA has proposed that all packaged foods bear this information.

Dietary fiber. Most cereals and other grain products list the fiber content, but the FDA will soon require this information on all food labels. Remember that 25 to 35 grams of dietary fiber is suggested for optimal health. Use the number of fiber grams listed to add up your daily total.

Sodium. The National Research Council recommends that we take in less than 2,400 milligrams daily. Use food labels to see how quickly sodium intake adds up. When buying packaged foods, compare sodium levels before you decide. For example, brands of frozen dinners vary in sodium content, so choose the one with the least.

Vitamins and minerals. The U.S. Recommended Daily Allowances (USRDA) for major vitamins and minerals are listed on food labels to help you make comparisons. This information helps you identify "empty" foods that provide little more than calories.

PLAYING IT SAFE

You gobble down a leftover take-out that's been in the fridge so long you don't remember putting it there. Do you ever wonder if it's still safe to eat? What about your suspicions concerning the safety of pesticides that might remain in the perfect-looking produce? If you worry at all, there are a few things you should know for safe Power Eating.

You must pay attention not only to the foods you select but also to the way you (or others) store and prepare them. While our nation's food supply is among the safest in the world, with pesticide and additive use strictly regulated, various government agencies and consumer groups say we need still tighter controls and tougher laws against pesticide residues in fresh fruits and vegetables and the contamination of chicken, eggs, and milk. But why wait for new legislation when *you* can protect yourself? Begin now to understand food safety issues and learn how to eat more safely.

HAZARD-FREE FEASTING

Eating doesn't have to be a high-risk activity; just follow these guidelines to widen the safety margin.

- ☐ Eat a variety of fresh, unprocessed foods.
- ☐ Rinse uncut fruits and vegetables before eating or cooking. (If you rinse them after they are cut or peeled, nutrients are washed away.)
- ☐ Peel fruits and vegetables coated with wax.
- ☐ Limit your intake of food dyes, found in artificially colored fruit drinks, candy, and commercial dessert items.
- ☐ Read food labels to determine additive use. (Note: Not all additives are required to be listed).
- ☐ Don't leave perishable foods out at room temperature for more than two hours.
- ☐ Rinse meat, poultry, and fish before cooking.
- ☐ Thoroughly wash all utensils and surfaces that come in contact with raw meats and poultry.
- ☐ Designate one cutting board (preferably plastic) for raw meats only.
- ☐ Cook eggs and poultry thoroughly.
- ☐ Cook the fish you eat to destroy parasites.

KITCHEN BASICS

Years ago, the kitchen was the heart of the household, filled with aromas of home cooking. Today's kitchens are more like command centers where ready-made or almost-ready-made foods are assembled and heated. Who cooks, except for holidays and special weekends? With our high-speed lifestyle, real cooking has been sacrificed in the time crunch. But good eating is still possible if you have a properly stocked kitchen; Power Foods can be ready in minutes, even seconds! Let me show you:

- ☐ How to get the most out of your microwave.
- ☐ What noncooks need as "cooking" utensils or gadgets.
- ☐ Which Power Foods to keep stocked in your cupboard.

Whether you're feeding just yourself or a family, you can put

together meals in minutes that will satisfy your taste and boost
your performance.

POWER EATING MAGIC
WITH YOUR MICROWAVE

Four out of five households have at least one microwave oven,
and many have a second for still more time savings and efficiency.
Despite the microwave's versatility, most people simply use it
to reheat cold pizza or to thaw out frozen meat. The microwave
can do much more for you. Learn to take full advantage of its
possibilities as an aid in your Power Eating efforts. It can be one
of the best tools you have to keep you on the fast track.

MICROWAVE SAFETY

How safe is the microwave—for the operator and the food?
There is still some question about how microwaving affects the
nutritional quality of foods compared to conventional cooking
methods. And new concerns center around chemicals, used in
special packaging for some commercial products, that could
leach into the food as it cooks.

Microwave cooking itself is safe and energy efficient. During
microwaving, electromagnetic waves are emitted inside the
oven, causing the water in food molecules to vibrate. That vibra-
tion generates heat in much the same way as two sticks that are
rubbed together to make fire.

The microwaves themselves penetrate only part of the food,
and the vibrating food molecules cook its interior. Electromagnetic rays dissipate completely and rapidly after emission has
stopped. Because vibrating food molecules continue the cooking
process after the electromagnetic waves have stopped, standing
time is necessary for certain foods.

Don't associate "nuking" the food with nuclear power plants.
Microwaves are in no way related to nuclear radiation and do
not cause any harmful mutations in you or the food. The waves
pass harmlessly through nonmetal cooking dishes and utensils.
(Remember, the rays can't penetrate metal, so metal cookware
can't be used.)

Contamination of your food with chemicals from certain microwave packaging, however, does pose a health concern. Many

packaging materials, such as plastics and special "heat-susceptors" designed to crisp foods, may give off chemicals that migrate into the foods during the cooking process. Some suspect these chemicals of causing cancer in laboratory animals, and they do migrate into the food in amounts that depend upon how hot the food becomes and how long the packaging is in contact with the food, both during and after cooking. Microwave-safe cookware may also present a chemical migration problem. The FDA does not regulate the cookware, or the plastic wrap you may put on your food while it's in the microwave, against potential chemical migration into food.

Glass is considered the perfect microwave cookware because there is virtually no transfer of chemicals from the glass to your food. Plastic tubs that once held margarine or yogurt, on the other hand, are best avoided, as these containers can readily transfer plastics to your food.

BETTER NUTRITION

As for nutritional damage to foods, microwave cooking causes minimal nutrient destruction. Microwaving your food destroys fewer nutrients than cooking by conventional methods such as boiling, baking, or frying. Since microwave cooking exposes foods to heat for a shorter period of time and because less water is used with microwave cooking than with conventional methods, more nutrients are preserved.

Certain vitamins—particularly vitamin C and thiamin—are destroyed by heat, so they actually benefit from the abbreviated microwave cooking times. Water-soluble nutrients, such as B vitamins and minerals, tend to leach out into cooking water, but microwave cooking is "waterless" for many vegetables and fruits, so the foods retain not only the water-soluble vitamins but more potassium and magnesium than those that are boiled.

HOT MICROWAVE TIPS

To maximize the performance of your microwave, first look over your machine's instruction manual for a refresher on waving. Most include suggested cooking times for various foods, based on your oven's power settings. Generally, the larger the volume of food being cooked, the longer the cooking time.

Microwave cooking is very versatile—you can use it to put together a quick snack in seconds or present an elaborate five-course gourmet meal quicker than by any other cooking method. Learn to use your microwave for timesaving, high-powered eating. Here are some tips:

Reheat leftovers for a quick but nutritious meal. Yesterday's spaghetti or last night's unfinished take-out makes a great power meal in the microwave. When you put together a low-fat lasagna or a casserole, make extra for quick microwave meals later in the week.

Low-fat main dish possibilities are endless. You can poach fish alongside a vegetable in six to eight minutes. Use spices such as tarragon or dill or specialty mustards to enhance the taste. Treat chicken or other poultry the same way, though cooking time is generally longer for poultry.

Beef can be cooked quickly for a low-fat main dish. Simply crumble lean ground beef in a microwave dish and drain the fat after cooking. You can use the cooked beef in soft tacos, casseroles, or soups, or mix it with ready-made pasta sauce.

Long-cooking vegetables are ready in minutes with a microwave. Nutrient-packed winter squash or spaghetti squash, along with potatoes or yams, cook in six to nine minutes. Topped with low-fat yogurt and fresh herbs, a combination of these vegetables makes a great high-carbohydrate main dish.

High-carbohydrate meal add-ons or snacks are quick to fix in a microwave. Heat flour or corn tortillas in a damp paper towel to accompany your favorite Mexican meal. Revive not-so-fresh breads, bagels, and muffins in seconds to serve with vegetable soup or a casserole.

Keep nutrient-packed frozen vegetables on hand as part of your Power Diet plan. They make a quick side dish, a welcome ingredient for casseroles or pasta dishes, or a tasty topping for microwaved potatoes or yams. Flavor frozen vegetables with herbs or a little balsamic vinegar before microwaving.

Microwavable snacks make great anytime high-carbohydrate eating. Popcorn designed for the microwave (make sure to choose an unbuttered version—check the label for fat grams) or frozen soft pretzels are great snacks for eating at home or to use in the microwave at work.

ESSENTIAL KITCHEN TOOLS

Whether you cook frequently or classify yourself as a "noncook," you need a few basic tools. My approach calls for simplicity in cooking gear. I don't have time to fuss with exotic kitchen gadgets; they only seem to end up getting lost in my kitchen "junk" drawer.

Beyond the standard refrigerator/freezer in every kitchen, here are some key appliances, cookware, and utensil needs for the Power Kitchen.

- □ *Microwave oven* equipped with rack and thermometer
- □ Basic set of *microwave cookware* that includes a compartmentalized dinner plate for reheating leftovers
- □ *Small food processor* (left out on the counter for easy use) for chopping vegetables to use in stir-fries, soups, salads, sauces, and the like
- □ *Blender* for soups, sauces, and blender drinks (see number 8 in "Ten Power Breakfast Suggestions" on page 255 for recipe)
- □ *Electric juicer* (attachment to food processor) for fresh fruit juice anytime
- □ *Nonstick pots and skillets* (one- and two-quart pots and 8- and 12-inch skillets) for cooking without added fats or oils
- □ *Plastic cooking utensils* (spoon, fork, spatula)
- □ *Vegetable and bread knives* (kept sharp)
- □ *Cheese slicer* to help slice cheese thin
- □ Set of *clear plastic storage containers* for keeping open packages of pasta, rice, cereal, and crackers fresh

Frozen and shelf-top meals are simple to fix. Serve them with a fresh green salad and a high-carbohydrate meal add-on like pita bread or a microwaved "baked" potato, and you have a great power meal. Check Table 10-1 for meals low in fat and sodium. Remember to select those that contain less than ten grams of fat and about 800 to 1,000 milligrams of sodium per meal.

BASIC STAPLES

Keep these staples on hand and replenish them when you shop so you always have the makings of a complete Power Meal.

In the Cupboard

- ☐ Two types of pasta
- ☐ Jar of spaghetti sauce
- ☐ Canned water-packed tuna
- ☐ Canned crushed tomatoes
- ☐ Tomato sauce
- ☐ Ready-to-eat breakfast cereal
- ☐ Quick-cooking oatmeal
- ☐ Package of low-fat cookies
- ☐ Quick-cooking brown rice
- ☐ Canned clams
- ☐ Canned refried beans
- ☐ Canned kidney beans
- ☐ Low-fat crackers like Ak-Mak or RyKrisp
- ☐ Small cans of vegetable juice
- ☐ Potatoes (store properly)

In the Refrigerator

- ☐ Low-fat or nonfat yogurt
- ☐ Parmesan cheese
- ☐ Eggs
- ☐ Broccoli
- ☐ Low-fat cheese
- ☐ Low-fat cottage cheese
- ☐ Carrots
- ☐ Oranges

In the Freezer

- ☐ Two types of vegetables (broccoli, spinach, cauliflower)
- ☐ Two loaves of whole-grain bread
- ☐ Orange and grapefruit juice concentrate
- ☐ Chicken thigh or breast fillets
- ☐ Three or four frozen complete dinners (check Table 10-1 for best selection)

(continued)

Staples—*Continued*

- ☐ Three or four frozen main dishes that allow you to add rice, veggies
- ☐ Fruit sorbet or frozen yogurt
- ☐ Frozen fruit (peaches, strawberries)

Spices and Extra Ingredients to Flavor Your Meals

- ☐ No-salt spices like Mrs. Dash
- ☐ Flavored and balsamic vinegars
- ☐ Cajun seasonings
- ☐ Fresh garlic/onions (and garlic and onion powders)
- ☐ Specialty mustards
- ☐ Olive or canola oil
- ☐ Worchestershire sauce
- ☐ Variety of dried herbs
- ☐ Fresh pepper grinder

Single-serve microwavable meals are a must to have on hand for busy schedules. You can even feed your family in shifts with these nutritious meals. (Check the label for fat and sodium.)

Dried fruits are packed with power nutrients and make great additions to salads, fruit compotes, or cereals. Plump up dried fruit by lightly sprinkling it with water. Cover and microwave on full power for about 30 seconds. Let the fruit stand about a minute, then add to your favorite dish.

KITCHEN NECESSITIES FOR POWER EATING

You don't have to be a chef to put together a Power Meal. With the right kitchen utensils and a properly stocked kitchen, anyone can do it anytime. Refer to "Essential Kitchen Tools" and "Basic Staples" on pages 279 and 280 for a list of what you need.

Now you know how to shop for, store, and prepare all the Power Foods you need to keep your performance at its peak. The rest is up to you.

INDEX